Precision Exercises

Precision Exercises

Exercises to Relieve Pain, Restore Posture, Improve Balance, and Regain Control of Muscles and Movement Needed for Everyday Living

by Brian P. Lambert, P.T.
B.L. Enterprises, LLC
Charlottesville, Virginia

The material presented in this book is not intended to be a substitute for direct and personal, professional medical care and opinion. To reduce the risk of injury, none of the exercises or activities mentioned in this book should be performed without clearance from your physician.

Exercise is not without its risks, and the exercises contained in this book, or other exercises, may result in injury.

The information in this book is in no way intended to replace or to be construed as medical advice and is offered for informational purposes only. As with any exercise, if you begin to feel faint, dizzy, or have physical discomfort, you should stop immediately and consult a physician. The information contained in this book should not be considered complete, nor should it be relied on to suggest a course of treatment for a particular individual. It should not be used in place of a visit, call, consultation or the advice of your physician or other qualified health care provider. Should you have any health care related questions, call or see your physician or other qualified health care provider promptly.

Reliance by you on any information contained in this book is solely at your own risk, and the author assumes no liability or responsibility for damage or injury to persons or property arising from your use of any information, idea, or instruction contained in this book.

Table of Contents

Acknowledgments

I wish to acknowledge the assistance of my family, friends, and colleagues who helped make this book possible. A special thanks to my wife, Ann, for her love, support, and artwork.

Thanks to June Cleveland for transcription, Rhonda Roebuck for pictures, Don Fry for editing, Katherine Garstang for layout and design, and David Rubin for advice.

Many people have shaped my views on the musculoskeletal system. Mark Bookout, Edward Isaacs, Philip Greenman, Florence Kendall, and David Butler are just a few who have had the greatest influence.

I wish to acknowledge all of my special patients (and you know who you are) who provide me with challenge and encouragement on a daily basis.

Introduction

During my 20 years treating musculoskeletal problems, I have identified in my patients four to five deficits that usually result in pain in the spine and/or extremities. This pain usually results from a portion of the musculoskeletal system doing more work than it was designed to do.

Our bodies are efficiently designed as hunting and gathering machines. People who still hunt and gather don't have problems with their neck, back, and extremities that we face in a modern society. These people use the body as it was designed to be used. Only in the last one to two hundred years have we become a more sedentary society. With increased education, computers, automobiles, and video games, we spend much more time sitting. **Sitting is a negative exercise.** It is worse than no exercise at all, because it creates most of the problems that lead to abnormal mechanics and improper motor patterns suffered by people in today's society.

The musculoskeletal system must be viewed as an integrated system. All of the components depend on one another. Any component that is not being used optimally shifts work to another area. When four or five components are not optimally used, a great deal of work gets shifted elsewhere.

Chronic musculoskeletal problems probably start developing the first day we enter kindergarten. At that time, we begin using the largest muscles we own as seat cushions, and we begin slumping forward. This combination leads to many problems. With proper reprogramming of the musculoskeletal system, many of these problems can be alleviated. This book contains the exercises I use on a daily basis with my patients. Most of them experience a significant degree of improvement just by doing the exercises alone. Manual therapy by a qualified professional will help optimize motion in restricted joints and accelerate recovery from a musculoskeletal problem.

The exercises in this book derive from many sources. Many of them were designed in response to the needs of a specific patient. When they worked well, they were then tried with other patients. If an exercise worked well enough, often enough, it was incorporated into an exercise program.

Much of my physical therapy training involved learning the principles of exercise for both orthopedic and neurological rehabilitation. In continuing education programs, the faculty of Michigan State University's School of Osteopathic Medicine emphasizes combining the principles of each area for musculoskeletal problems. There are exercises in this book taken directly from their course work. There are other exercises, whose sources I cannot recall, that are neither original nor from Michigan State Programs.

I hope you can use these exercises to stay pain free and functional throughout your lifetime.

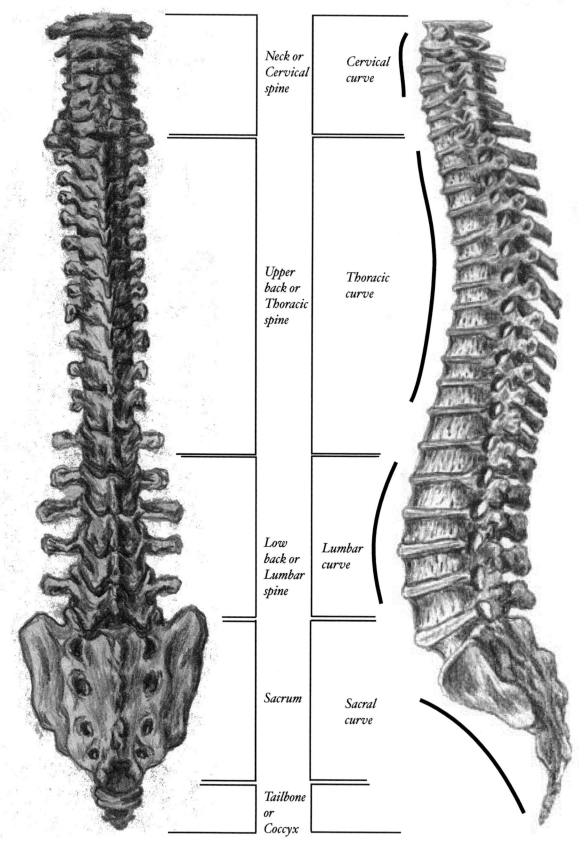

Neck or
Cervical
spine

Cervical
curve

Upper
back or
Thoracic
spine

Thoracic
curve

Low
back or
Lumbar
spine

Lumbar
curve

Sacrum

Sacral
curve

Tailbone
or
Coccyx

Spine from rear

Spine from left side

BONES OF THE BACK

ANATOMY

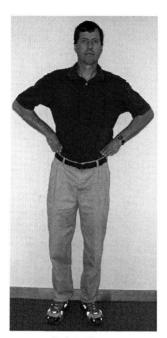

Pelvic Bones

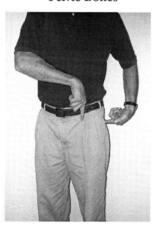

Hip Joint

This book deals mainly with the spine, pelvis, and shoulders. Place your hands over your waist. Your hands come into contact with the pelvic bones. A little below that, we have the hip bones. Inside the hip bones are the ball and socket that make up the hip joint. The socket is part of the pelvis. The top of the thigh bone or femur is made up of the hip bone and the ball portion of the hip joint. The bottom of the femur is the top half of the knee. There is a wedge bone between the pelvic bones called the sacrum. The sacrum is composed of five fused vertebrae. They generally fuse from individual vertebrae by the time we reach our late teens. The sacrum is connected to the pelvic bone by sacroiliac joints. These joints are tied to the pelvis by very strong ligaments from the front and the back. The pelvic bones are joined in the front at the pubic symphysis, which is also tied together with ligaments.

The spine is composed of individual bones called vertebra. Just above the sacrum, the bottom five vertebrae make up the lumbar spine. Where the ribs attach, we have 12 thoracic vertebrae. Most of our ribs attach between the thoracic vertebrae. The seven cervical vertebrae are located between the base of the skull and the bottom of the neck.

The blocks of bone that make up the front of most vertebrae are called vertebral bodies The vertebral bodies are separated by discs. The discs are very much like high performance jelly doughnuts. The inside of the disc is called a nucleus and has the consistency of crabmeat. The outside of the disc is called the annulus and is very much like automobile tire material. The annulus is very strong, but, over time, it can be worn down and ruptured if subjected to chronic overload. The discs provide multi-directional movement in the spine. They are not designed to act as shock absorbers.

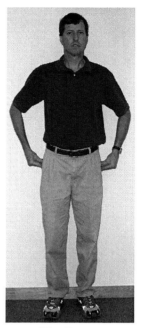

Hip Bones

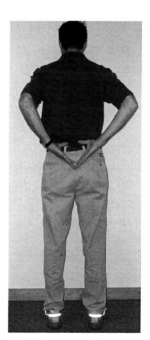

The Sacrum is between the pelvic bones.

On the back of the spine, there are joints called facet joints. Facet joints link the vertebrae together. The surfaces of the facet joints are lined with cartilage. A joint capsule surrounds them. Inside the joint capsule, the synovial membrane secretes synovial fluid into the joint. As the surface of one facet moves over the surface of another the synovial fluid helps provide nutrition and lubrication to the cartilage. The facet joints stand at difference angles in different parts of the spine. The orientation of the facet joints will determine the kind of movement allowed in a given section of the spine.

The whole spinal column is bound with very strong ligaments that hold it together but allow movement. Bone spurs may occur where the ligaments attach to the bone as a result of continuous stress on that attachment.

MECHANICAL CONSIDERATIONS

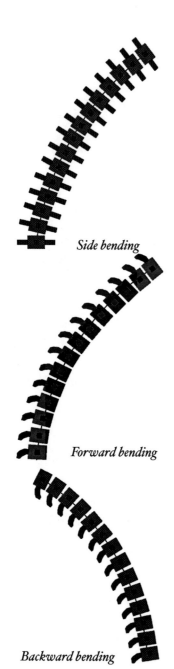

Side bending

Forward bending

Backward bending

One of the first things to observe in the spine and pelvis is how well everything moves. Motion in any direction should be uniform from the bottom of the sacrum to the top of the neck. All of the vertebrae should move like links in a chain. Since life activities tend to bend us forward, the thoracic spine and sacrum become stuck in some degree of forward bending or "flexion." To achieve upright posture, we tend to bend backward or over-extend through the low back and neck. "Hypermobility" occurs when there is too much motion between two or more vertebrae. Hypermobility is probably responsible for arthritis or other degeneration commonly seen in the lower lumbar and lower cervical portions of the spine.

Mechanics of the sacrum and pelvis can be very confusing. If mechanics are good, forward bending of the trunk causes the top of the sacrum to move backwards and the bottom of the sacrum to move forward. The opposite motions occur with bending backward. Imagine two stacked cereal boxes. If the top box falls over in one direction, the bottom box tends to fall in the opposite direction. The bottom cereal box represents the sacrum. The sacral motion between the pelvic bones occurs until the slack is taken up in the ligaments, then the pelvic bones move with the trunk. The first few degrees of forward or backward motion should be isolated to the spine and sacrum.

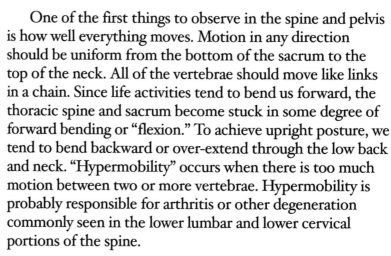

Sacral motion between the pelvic bones

Backward bending   *Neutral*   *Forward bending*

The mechanics of the pelvis and spine become more complicated when we walk or run. One side of the pelvis is rotating with the lead leg. The other side of the pelvis is rotating with the trailing leg in the opposite direction. This generally causes a slight bit of rotation and sidebending in the spine and sacrum. Everything, the spine, sacrum, and pelvic bones, must move freely. One of the most common mechanical problems in the pelvis occurs when the top of the sacrum on one side is pushed back and stuck. The lack of motion in the sacroiliac joint is called "mechanical dysfunction." Adaptation higher up in the spine contributes to increased work in the low back. The mechanical dysfunction also affects the pelvic bone. Since the hip socket is part of the pelvic bone, extra work may be transmitted to the hip joint, then to the knee, then to the foot.

In the musculoskeletal system, a deficit in one area increases the workload in another area. This principle applies to the hip joints. Restriction of mobility will increase workload of the spine, pelvis, and legs.

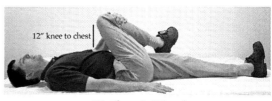

Good mobility of the hips should allow you to pull your leg towards the center of the chest to within 12 inches of your chest. A tight piriformis muscle deep in the buttock will restrict this movement. Inward rotation of the hips should allow you to sit in a chair with your knees and thighs together and your feet 18 to 20 inches apart. Good outward rotation would allow the shin of one leg to be parallel to the floor when the ankle is placed on the opposite knee. Restrictions in rotation of the thighbone may be due to tightness of the muscles at the hip joint or arthritic changes in the hip joint.

Hip extension is the movement of the thigh behind the body when we walk. Good hip extension should allow you to lie face down and have someone lift your leg so that the knee is 8 to 12 inches off the surface without causing movement at the pelvis. Tight hip flexors muscles can restrict this movement.

Piriformis Muscle

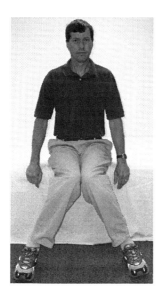

Inward rotation of hip

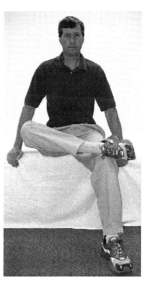

Outward rotation of hip

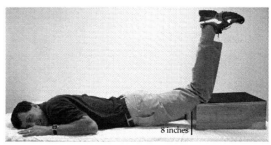

Hip extension

POSTURE

Several components must be in place for good posture. Essentially all of the parts must be stacked one on top of another, very much like a building in which all the walls are plumb. If all our components are stacked one on top of another, the bones hold us up, not the muscles. The main function of the muscles is to control movement of our body. Good posture generally involves having the ears over the shoulders, the shoulders over the hips, and the hips over the ankles.

The benefits of good posture are many. First, all of the spinal segments are in a completely neutral position. A neutral position of the vertebrae means that the bottom surface of the vertebra is parallel to the top surface of the vertebra below it. Loading is then distributed evenly across the disc, which is sandwiched between the vertebral bodies. Another benefit of neutral position of the vertebrae involves a phenomenon known as Fryette's law, which generally states that if motion is taken up in one direction, there is less motion available in other directions. A segment that starts from a neutral position has maximum motion available in any single direction. When you turn your head or trunk, each segment should move uniformly, like links in a chain. Stress of movement will then be evenly distributed. But out-of-neutral segments cause a "kink" in the system, and stress increases above and below the kink.

When all of the segments are in neutral positions, the spine has four primary curves. Generally there is some sway or "lordosis" to the low back and neck. There is a forward curvature or "kyphosis" through the thoracic spine as well as through the sacrum and pelvis. Like a spring, the neutral curves allow movement that will provide for shock absorption. If there is too little curve in the back, a great deal of compressive force is driven straight down, especially through the lower vertebrae. If there is too much curve, as with a sway back, then shearing forces develop.

There are many adaptations to poor posture. Some of these involve severe retraction of the head and neck, flattening of the lumbar spine, or severe forward sway to the pelvis. Too often mechanics in one area are sacrificed to compensate for problems in another. If you don't stand up straight, your muscles work too hard and cause problems.

GOOD POSTURE

Good Posture

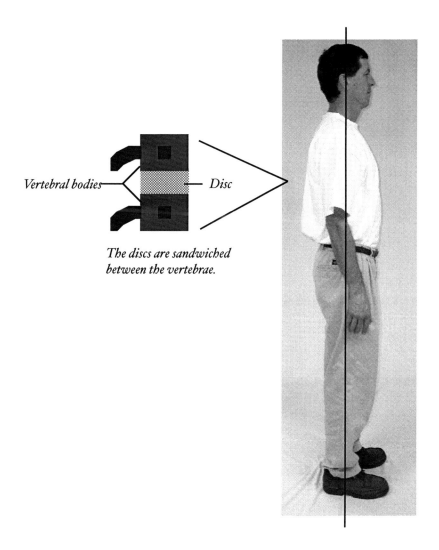

Vertebral bodies — *Disc*

The discs are sandwiched between the vertebrae.

MUSCLES OF THE HIPS AND PELVIS

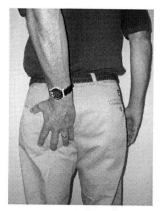

Gluteus Maximus Muscle

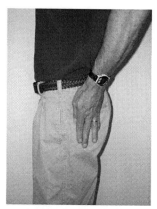

Gluteus Medius and
Minimus Muscles

The muscles located in your buttock area are the most important muscles in the body for control, balance, and motion. The largest muscles in your body are located there. The "tush" can be thought of as the keystone of the musculoskeletal system. It is the main propulsion unit. It is the foundation the spine sits on. It is the main area for control of balance.

The entire buttock area is a package of muscles. The largest muscle in the body is the gluteus maximus. This muscle is a hip extensor and attaches along the pelvis and sacrum and crosses the hip joint to attach to the upper portion of the thighbone. Ahead of this muscle, but behind and above the hipbone, are the gluteus medius and gluteus minimus muscles. These large muscles are commonly called hip abductors. Long periods of sitting will alter how well we can activate or "recruit" the gluteus maximus, medius, and minimus muscles when we move. These muscles are usually very weak and not well recruited. Underneath the gluteus maximus are the smaller hip rotators. These include the piriformis, the gemelli superior, gemelli inferior, quadratus femoris, obturator internus, and obturator externus (not pictured). All of these muscles surround the center of gravity of the body. The most efficient way to control an object is at its center of gravity. One side of the tush muscles must be strong enough to lift and control the entire weight of the body. This must happen with every step you take.

Tightness or inflexibility in muscles should be viewed as an adaptation to overuse. The spring on a garage door reduces the energy you must expend to open the door manually. A tight muscle is spring-loaded and becomes much more energy efficient. The same phenomenon occurs with young men who lift very heavy weights on a repetitive basis. They become "muscle bound." This term refers not only to their bulkiness, but also to their lack of mobility. If you lose too much mobility in a muscle, then the tightness itself becomes a problem. The large muscles in the hip tend to be very weak. The muscles that can substitute for them will tend to be overused and become very tight. The hamstrings, on the back of the thigh, are secondary hip extensors but mainly control the knee. If the hamstrings have to do both jobs constantly, full-time, they will get tight. The smaller hip rotators can substitute to some degree for the hip abductors and extensors, and will also tend to get very tight. The low back muscles can substitute to some degree for the hip abductors, and again will get very tight if they are overused on a chronic basis. The tightness in these muscles will not be alleviated until the large muscles are not only strong, but are also activated or "recruited" appropriately when you move.

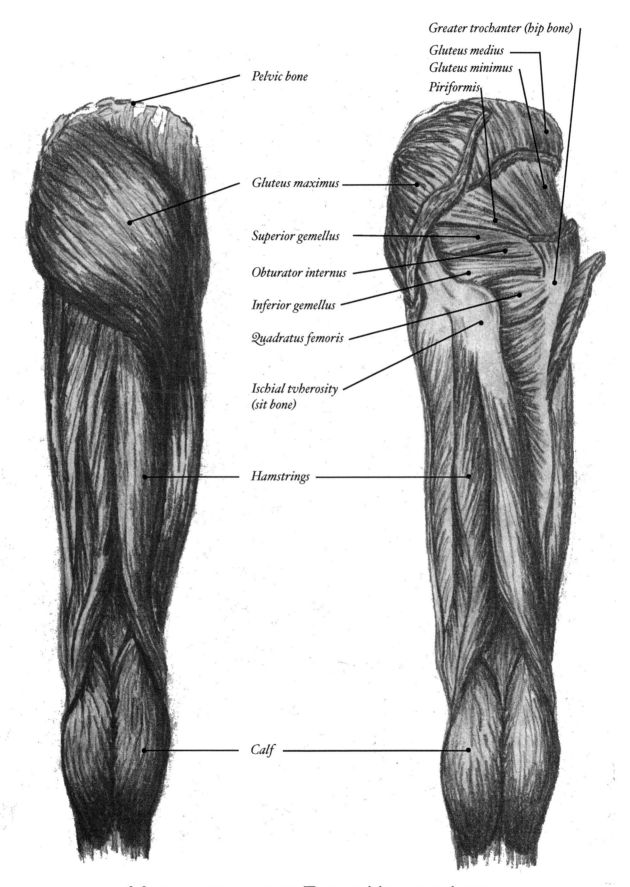

Greater trochanter (hip bone)

Gluteus medius

Gluteus minimus

Piriformis

Pelvic bone

Gluteus maximus

Superior gemellus

Obturator internus

Inferior gemellus

Quadratus femoris

Ischial tvherosity
(sit bone)

Hamstrings

Calf

MUSCLES OF THE RIGHT HIP AND LEG

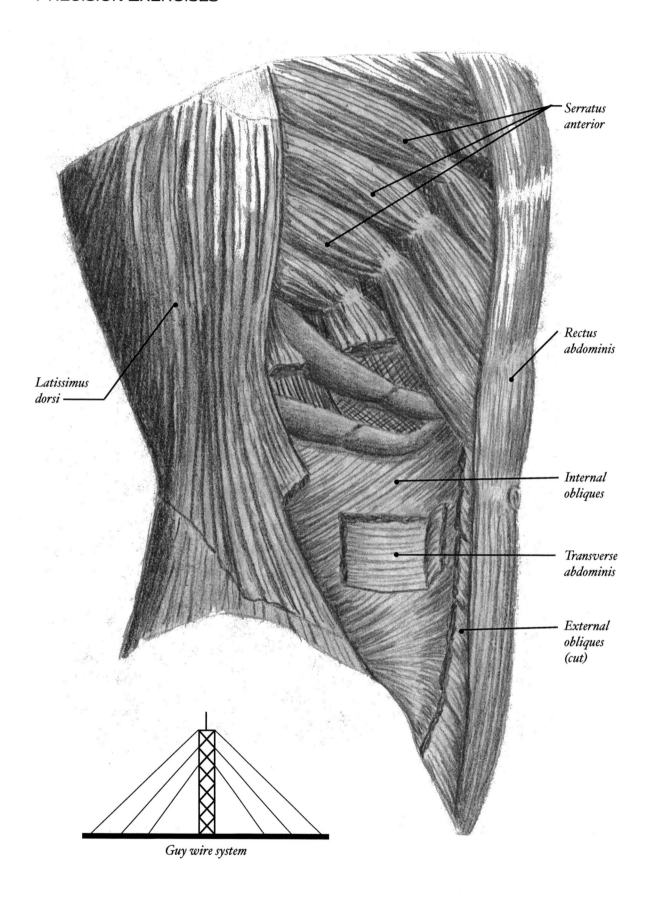

Serratus anterior

Rectus abdominis

Latissimus dorsi

Internal obliques

Transverse abdominis

External obliques (cut)

Guy wire system

MUSCLES OF THE GUY-WIRE SYSTEM

Muscles of the Guy-Wire System

The muscles that wrap around the body from the rib cage down to the pelvis represent a guy-wire system. An example of a guy-wire system would be the cable supports that hold up radio antennas. The tension in these wires must balance out so the antenna is evenly supported. Likewise, there must be a dynamic control through muscles of the trunk. In the front and sides, these muscles include the rectus abdominis, internal and external obliques, transverse abdominis, and the hip flexors (not pictured). More around the back lie the erector spinae, quadratus lumborum, and to some degree, the latissimus dorsi. These muscles must be trained and strengthened as guy-wires. Activities such as sit ups, curls, crunches, and flexion machines tend to train and strengthen the muscles incorrectly and may worsen posture by increasing forward bending or flexion through the thoracic spine. The abdominal musculature is mainly used in a sit-up motion when getting out of bed. During upright movements this musculature needs to be used as part of the guy-wire system.

Many people have gross imbalance and lack of control in these muscles. Activation of each of these opposing muscle groups should be as easy as using the biceps and triceps in the upper arm when bending and straightening the elbow.

Neck, Upper Back, and Shoulders

Most of the problems with pain in the neck and shoulders can be traced back to poor positioning and/or movement patterns. There is usually muscle imbalance in the neck, upper back, and rib cage. Forward head posture occurs when the thoracic spine is stuck in a flexed position, and the head is in front of the shoulders. Your head weighs as much as a bowling ball. If a bowling ball must be carried in an upright position, it is best kept centered and balanced. If you allow the bowling ball to tip forward, more muscle effort is required to keep it in place. More muscle effort is required with forward head posture.

Postural muscles in the front of the neck include the scalene and deep neck flexors. One end of the scalene muscles attaches along the sides of the vertebrae of the neck, and the other end attaches to the first and second ribs just behind the collarbones. The deep neck flexors attach to the front of the vertebra of the neck. Forward head posture causes overuse of the scalenes and underuse of the deep neck flexors.

The deep muscles along the upper back and back of the neck include the various layers of the spinal extensors or erector spinae. These muscles can attach from one vertebra to the next, from vertebra to the skull, or from rib cage to the vertebra. The more shallow muscles of the back include the trapezius, levator scapulae, and rhomboids. One end of these muscles attaches to the shoulder blade and the other end attaches to the spine. The upper portion of the trapezius attaches to the back of the head.

Forward head posture will cause overuse of the upper trapezius, levator scapula, and erector spinae in the neck, and underuse of the thoracic erector spinae, rhomboids, and the lower portion of the trapezius. Overused muscles will become tight and painful. Underused muscles will become weak and poorly recruited. Good posture involves keeping the ears over the shoulders, the shoulders over the hips, and the hips over the ankles. This lineup will encourage optimal usage of all of the postural musculature.

The arms are basically slung onto the spine and rib cage with a series of supportive muscles, generally called "scapular stabilizers." Included in this group are the trapezius musculature, serratus anterior, rhomboids, pectoralis minor (not pictured), and levator scapula. All of these muscles attach from the spine or rib cage to the shoulder blade. The trapezius and levator musculature do double duty. One end helps support the head and neck. The other end is attached to the shoulder blade to help control and stabilize the shoulder. If posture is poor, too much of their work is devoted to controlling the head and neck, and less control is available to the shoulder. The latissimus dorsi and pectoralis or chest musculature attach to the upper arm and then to the rib cage and spine. If posture is poor, these muscles can become tight and adversely affect shoulder function.

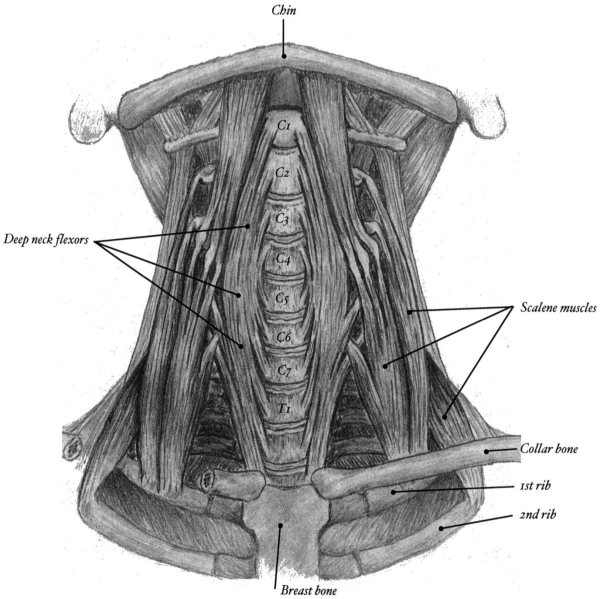

POSTURAL MUSCLES IN THE FRONT OF THE NECK

The rotator cuff muscles attach to the shoulder blade and then to the upper portion of the arm. Their primary purpose is to control movement in the ball and socket that make up the shoulder or "glenohumeral joint." The socket is part of the shoulder blade, and the ball is part of the bone of the upper arm. Movement in the ball and socket accounts for only a portion of the total movement available to the arm. If you start with your arm at your side and raise it up so that it is pointing straight up over your head, only half of this motion occurs in the "shoulder joint." The other half is the shoulder blade moving on the rib cage. Positioning and control of the socket and rotator cuff muscles is dependent on the scapular stabilizers, which are dependent on how well the spine and rib cage function. Good functioning of the spine and rib cage usually depends on good posture. Less than optimal control of the shoulder blade leads to shoulder problems.

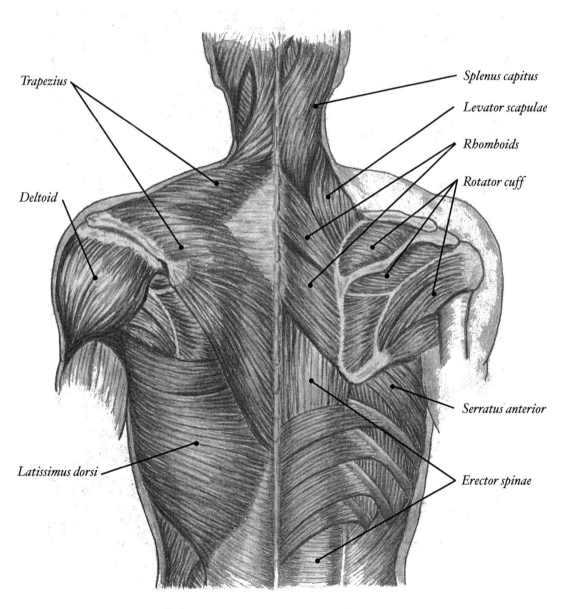

Trapezius

Splenus capitus

Levator scapulae

Rhomboids

Rotator cuff

Deltoid

Serratus anterior

Latissimus dorsi

Erector spinae

MUSCLES OF THE BACK
DEEP MUSCLES ON RIGHT SIDE

BEFORE YOU BEGIN

Our bodies are not designed for static positioning or repetitive motion. Sitting can be viewed as a negative exercise. We were not designed for prolonged sitting because it creates tremendous pressure on the buttock muscles. This area is not designed as a seat cushion. Sitting would be the same as asking someone to sit on their hand for 15 or 20 minutes. The hand would not be of much use until the circulation and feeling returned. This happens to the buttock area every day. Theoretically, if you sat long enough you would kill the skin and muscle tissue and subsequently develop a pressure sore. The gluteal area is designed in such a redundant fashion that we can learn to do without the large muscles for an extended period of time. Over years, the work of the gluteals is transferred up to the back, into the piriformis muscle, and down to the knees and ankles, causing problems. Not using your big muscle causes big pain elsewhere.

Sitting also increases forward bending of the mid and upper back, which leads to a worsening posture problem. The skeletal system out of plumb alters how the guy-wire muscle system works. Once we have adopted abnormal movement patterns, it is difficult to unlearn them without specific exercises designed to activate or "recruit" muscles that are no longer used on a regular basis.

Most of the exercises described in this book deal with reprogramming the body so that we can optimally distribute the workload of everyday life evenly over the musculoskeletal system. All of these exercises must be done carefully with specific attention to the target of each exercise. **You should consult with your physician, physical therapist, and/or trainer to be sure you can do these exercises safely and effectively.**

Some of the trunk exercises are done in two phases. The early retraining is done in an "open kinetic chain" exercise, with one end of the leg off the ground. The later phase is a "closed kinetic chain," with one end of the leg fixed, usually on the ground.

An example of an open kinetic chain exercise would be lying on your side and lifting your leg as in a side leg lift. A squat is an example of a closed kinetic chain exercise. Our propulsion and support muscles are designed to work in the closed kinetic chain mode. It is very important to be able to recruit these muscles with the foot on the ground.

AVOID PAIN

Pain is the body's signal that something is wrong. With the musculoskeletal system, it is often the last indicator of a problem. If a problem starts gradually or without a precipitating event, or if there is an injury that does not resolve, then part of the body is probably working too hard.

Exercises or other activities that cause pain are only reinforcing non-optimal muscle activation or recruitment patterns. When something hurts, you are placing strain on an area that does not need more strain. Consider a blister on the palm of your hand from too much raking or shoveling. When that area is raw and angry, the last thing you want to do is rub or irritate it in any way. Musculoskeletal pain is basically "a blister" or raw spot on the inside of the body. Causing more hurt in that area would be the same as bothering an irritated place on your palm. Don't do it: causing pain won't get rid of pain.

1
Basic Low Back Exercises

The basic back set consists of five exercises. One exercise stretches the deep rotators of the hips. Three of these exercises are designed to reprogram the major supportive muscles in the trunk and the pelvis. The other is for postural retraining. There is no specific order in which the exercises should be done.

Each of the exercises has a purpose and a specific target. If you miss the target, the exercise is a waste of time. Your brain tells the body what muscles to use to make movements happen. Because the body is an adaptive, learning machine, this program can be altered. Learning a dance or other specific activity involves reprogramming or altering the body's movement program. You can start to change your motor program by doing the exercises as described.

Long periods of sitting are one of the worst positions for the body. The gluteal musculature gets smashed. The thoracic spine and sacrum get jammed into a flexed position. The abdominals are not needed. Repeated bouts of sitting (*i.e.* K through 12) will alter our motor program into a substitution program, which ultimately becomes our standard motor program.

In this substitution pattern, much of the work of balance, lift, and propulsion gets transferred to either the lower back or the legs. The low back musculature can get grossly overused and tight, leading to increased compressive forces and increased overall work done in the lower part of the lumbar spine. If the pelvis is shifted forward, the hip flexors and thighs become involved, leading to overuse of the hips, knees, ankles, and feet, as well as additional compressive force in the lower lumbar spine.

Runners and weekend warriors may transfer their work mostly to the legs and develop problems in those areas. Most people transfer the work to the lower back and therefore experience increased levels of low back pain.

The five basic beginning exercises are the supine piriformis stretch, prone gluteal retraining, clam, pelvic clock, and wall angel. Substitute exercises can be done if the primary exercise does not hit the target.

The muscular retraining exercises done lying down will prepare you for doing a stand-up version of muscle re-education. Your body doesn't need supportive muscles when you lie down. You only need them when you're vertical. Complete re-integration of a muscle group into upright movement won't take place until you activate or recruit the muscle during the activity for which it is designed. The gluteal muscles need to work when the foot is on the ground, and the guy-wires need to work when the trunk is vertical. Good posture makes little difference when the body is horizontal, but is a big factor when you're upright.

The lie-down exercises are important to help you learn to isolate a muscle or muscle group. They teach the brain where the muscle is. The stand-up exercises teach the brain how the muscle functions, and then you can reinforce the correct motor pattern as well as strengthen the muscle.

SUPINE PIRIFORMIS STRETCH

This exercise stretches the smaller hip rotators located deep in the buttock region. Start by lying on your back with the right thigh at 90 degrees to the floor and the left leg straight. Using the right hand, bring the right knee to the midline of the body. Grab the right shin with the left hand to rotate the lower portion of the leg across the body. Keep the knee in the centerline of the body, and then pull equally on the leg with both hands. Fine-tune by increasing or decreasing the amount of rotation and/or changing the positioning of the knee by slightly moving the knee to one side or the other. You should feel a sensation of gentle stretch in the buttock area. Occasionally you may feel some of the stretch down the back of the thigh. Hold the position for 15 seconds, and do 3 repetitions on each side. If pinching occurs in the groin area, move the leg to one side or the other. Do not pull so hard that the pelvis twists or you feel pain.

For a more aggressive stretch, try the quadriped version in the Stretches section (p. 61).

SUPINE PIRIFORMIS STRETCH

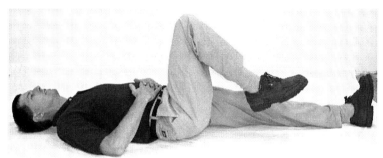

1. Lie on back.   Thigh 90 degrees.

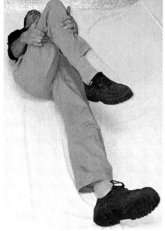

2. Bring the knee to the center of the chest.

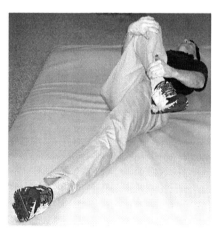

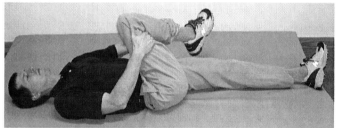

4. Pull the leg toward the chest to feel gentle stretch in buttock area. Adjust leg for best stretch with least movement. Search for the tightest spot.

3. Shin 30-40 degrees across the body.

Hold 15 seconds.
Do 3 on each side.

Avoid Pain!

THE CLAM

This exercise isolates and retrains the gluteus medius and gluteus minimus musculature, commonly called the hip abductors. These muscles are located behind and slightly above the hipbone, which positions them on either side of the center of gravity of the body. With one foot on the ground in a single leg stance, they keep the pelvis level and prevent the knee from rotating inward. They also provide a push to move us sideways.

The target of this exercise is just behind the top hipbone. Begin by lying on your side in a "hook lying" position. Put the thighs at 90 degrees to the trunk and the knees bent to approximately 120 degrees. Having your back against a wall or couch will keep the lower trunk from rotating and help improve recruitment of the gluteus medius and minimus. Keep your heels together and raise your top knee about three to four inches. Try several repetitions. If you're not hitting the target, bring your knees closer to the chest and try again. Sometimes less bend at the knees and hips will localize the work to the target area. If you're still having difficulty activating the muscle, follow a sequence of clenching the buttock muscle, then squeezing the heels together, then raising the knee. Start with 3 sets of 6 to 10 repetitions.

If you can't isolate the appropriate area with this exercise, then a side-lying hip raise or hydrant exercise (see next two exercises) will sometimes work. If none of these works the gluteus medius and minimus, move on to the gluteus maximus retraining for a week or so, then retry the clam exercise.

When this exercise gets very easy so that you can do 3 sets of 15 repetitions without strain, then progress to one of the closed chain exercises. These include side step lunge, single leg door frame squat, or ball on the wall exercise (pp. 38–43).

THE CLAM

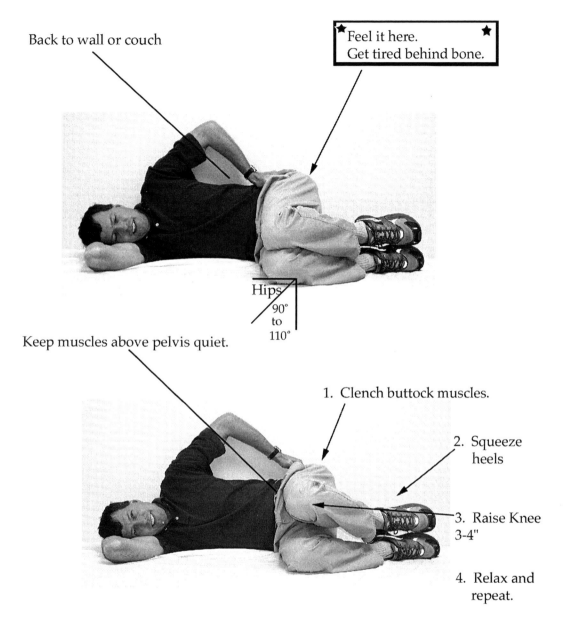

Back to wall or couch

Feel it here.
Get tired behind bone.

Hips
90°
to
110°

Keep muscles above pelvis quiet.

1. Clench buttock muscles.

2. Squeeze heels

3. Raise Knee 3-4"

4. Relax and repeat.

3 sets of 6-10 per side.
Rest 30 seconds between sets.

Avoid Pain!

SIDE-LYING LEG RAISE

This exercise is an attempt to isolate recruitment of the hip abductors. It's generally a second choice because other musculature is too easily used.

Try to keep the top thigh relaxed and the top foot turned slightly downward. Again, if the area of focus is not behind the hipbone, you may want to try a different exercise and wait until the musculature is better recruited.

Lie on your side with your back against a wall or front of a couch. Roll your pelvis slightly forward so that the top buttock cheek and shoulder are slightly away from the wall, but the heel of the top leg remains against the wall. The bottom leg may be slightly bent.

Before lifting the top leg, tighten the stomach muscles and push the top leg down and away from your body to elongate the top of the trunk. Point the toes of the top leg toward the floor. Now lift the top leg, keeping the top heel against the wall. Keep the muscles above the pelvis inactive as you raise the leg so that the foot is 6 to 8 inches from the floor. Lower the leg slowly and repeat the leg lift.

Side-lying Leg Raise

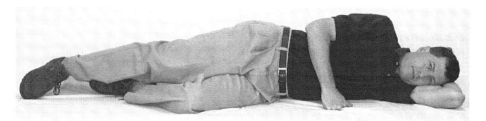

1. Lie on side, body in a straight line with back to front of couch. Bottom leg bent. Roll the pelvis slightly forward. Top cheek and shoulder away from couch; top heel in contact.

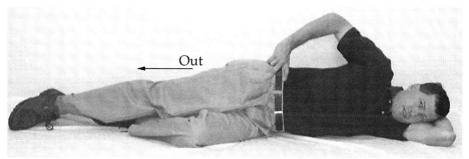

Out

2. Tighten the tummy slightly. Push the top leg "out".

Get tired behind hipbone.

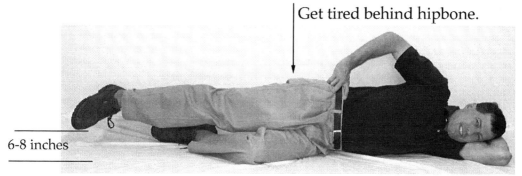

6-8 inches

3. Lift the top leg 6-8 inches. Keep the muscles above the pelvis quiet.

3 sets of 8-10 repetitions per side.
30 second rest between sets.

Avoid Pain!

HYDRANT EXERCISE

Do this exercise on all fours. While keeping the pelvis level, lift one leg to the side. By varying the forward or backward positioning or rotational movement of the leg, sometimes the reluctant abductors can be activated and isolated. For some people, this works better than the clam or side-lying hip abduction.

HYDRANT EXERCISE

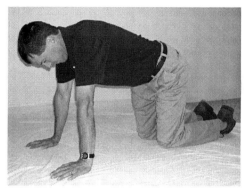

1. Starting position.

2. Raise leg to side.

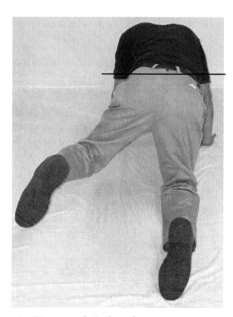

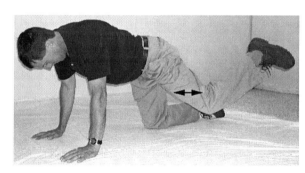

3. Adjust leg to find muscle behind hip bone.

4. Keep pelvis level.

3 sets of 8-10 repetitions per side.
30-second rest between sets.

Avoid Pain!

PRONE GLUTEAL RETRAINING

The gluteus maximus (your butt muscle) is the largest muscle in the body. To begin retraining this muscle, lie on your stomach with pillows under your pelvis and stomach. Bend both ankles so the tips of the toes touch the floor and the ankle is positioned at 90 degrees to the floor. Clench the buttock muscles only, and then straighten just one knee. Maintain gluteal contraction and slowly lift the whole leg only one inch. Point your toe as if you are pressing on a gas pedal, and then slowly lower the leg. Relax for a moment, and then do the same sequence on the other side. Usually 10 repetitions, 5 on each side, are sufficient.

Keep the exercise slow and controlled. Make sure that the knee remains locked when you lift. If the knee bends, the hamstring musculature will provide too much assistance. Lifting the leg too high or too fast will over-recruit the musculature in the low back.

Poor contraction of the gluteus maximus can be a problem. More pillows under the abdomen will help.

Some people will start the next exercise, the supine version, if isolated gluteal contraction is poor. If the muscles in front of the hip are tight, inhibition of the gluteal musculature may occur. It may be necessary to stretch these muscles before good contraction of the gluteus maximus can be obtained. If this exercise is done well, it should become very easy within 5 to 7 days. Occasionally patients take up to 3 weeks before they can progress to the closed chain exercises. See Advanced Hip Exercises, p. 33.

PRONE GLUTEAL RETRAINING

On tummy with 1 or 2 pillows under abdomen

Start with ankles bent.
1. Clench buttock muscles.

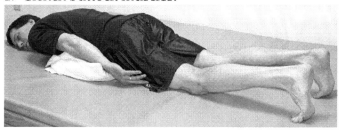

2. Straighten knee to locked position. Keep tight.

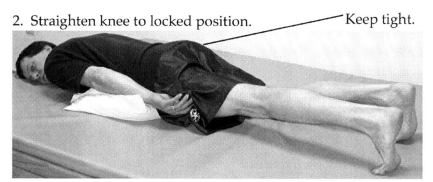

3. *Slowly*-lift whole leg just *1 inch*. Keep knee locked straight

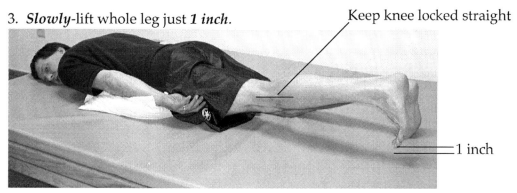

1 inch

4. Point the foot, then *lower slowly*. Relax buttock muscles.

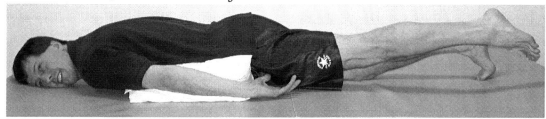

5. Retighten. Repeat sequence on the other side.

Do 10 total. 5 per side.

Avoid Pain!

SUPINE GLUTEAL RETRAINING

If the prone gluteal retraining exercise doesn't work well, the supine version may prove a better starting point to isolate and activate the gluteus maximus. This exercise can be done on a bed or on the floor.

Lie on your back with 2 to 3 pillows under your knees. Cup your hands around the buttock musculature on either side. Clench the buttock muscles only, and then use the buttock muscle to press one knee down into the pillows. Avoid tension in the thigh. Hold for 5 seconds. Emphasize pressing the leg down from the hip. You should feel an increase in the tension or firmness in the gluteal musculature on the active side. This exercise will teach the brain where the "butt" is. When this exercise becomes easy, then progress to the prone version of the gluteus maximus retraining (previous page).

SUPINE GLUTEAL RETRAINING

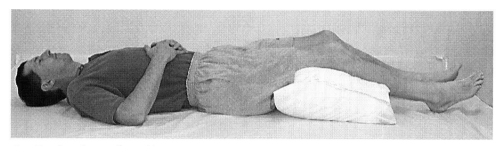

1. On back with pillows under your knees.

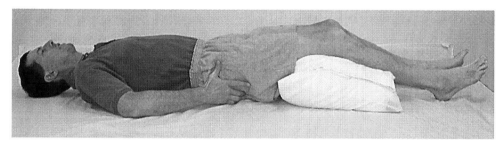

2. Clench buttock muscles.

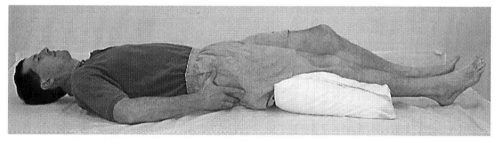

3. Press **ONE** knee down using the gluteal muscles. Hold 5 seconds.
Relax, retighten buttock muscles. Press the other knee down.
Do 5 per side for a total of 10.

Avoid Pain!

PELVIC CLOCK

The guy-wire system of muscles attaches from the rib cage to the pelvis, all around the torso. As we move, there should be a dynamic interplay among these groups of muscles.

The pelvic clock exercise begins the process of restoring control to this area. Crunches, curls, and sit-ups will strengthen the abdominal musculature, but they may also worsen posture, and do not necessarily teach good active control of the musculature.

The pelvic clock is done lying on your back with your legs propped up so they are well supported and can remain passive during the exercise. Grab the pelvis by resting the thumbs on the front of the pelvic bones with the fingers wrapped around the hips.

Visualize a clock resting on your tummy so that 12 o'clock is up towards your head and 6 o'clock is down towards your feet. Arch the low back only so that the front of the pelvis rotates upward towards the 6 o'clock direction. Keep the upper back, buttocks, and legs relaxed. If you find these areas are activated, reduce the amount of effort and motion until all of the work gets done in the low back, and the pelvis and low back are the only parts of the body that are moving.

The second step, the 12 o'clock tilt, uses the exact opposite motion of the 6 o'clock tilt. It should be done with the exact opposite muscle group: the abdominals. Begin the exercise by pulling the belly button in and up under the rib cage. This should cause the low back to flatten against the floor and the pelvis to rotate in a posterior or 12 o'clock direction. Again make sure the thighs, buttock, and chest are quiet. These are not part of the guy-wire system. You may rest your hands on your thighs during the exercise to monitor for increased tension. If you have difficulty keeping the thigh muscles relaxed, decrease the amount of pelvic movement.

Balance the musculature by doing a 6 o'clock tilt first, and hold for 5 seconds. Then as you relax out of the 6 o'clock tilt, immediately contract the abdominal musculature and hold the 12 o'clock tilt for 5 seconds. Relax for 5 seconds and then repeat. Usually a total of 5 to 6 repetitions are sufficient for a session. If you have a flat back and 6 o'clock is the difficult direction to initiate, then do 12 o'clock first, hold, then transition to 6 o'clock.

When the basic pelvic clock exercise is easy, try moving the pelvis back and forth from 5 o'clock to 11 o'clock several times. Now move to the 7 o'clock to 10'clock direction. The pelvic bones should move like a rolling pin when you're rolling out cookie dough. Moving smoothly through the diagonal patterns will help balance the guy-wire muscles.

PELVIC CLOCK

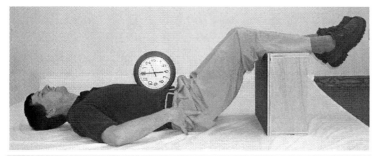

Start with relaxed pelvis and spine. Legs on a chair or stool.

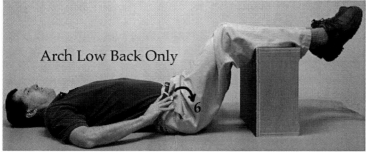

Arch Low Back Only

Gently arch into 6:00. Hold 5 seconds, relax.

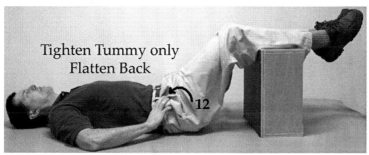

Tighten Tummy only
Flatten Back

Gently transition to 12:00. Hold 5 seconds.

Rest 5 seconds, then repeat sequence.

Do 5 repetitions.

If 12:00 is easier than 6:00 then reverse the sequence.

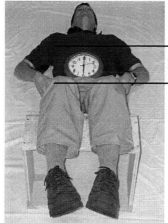

Keep Work Between Lines

Avoid Pain!

WALL ANGEL

Improvement in posture can be accomplished with the wall angel exercise. Keep in mind that posture happens all the way down to the ground. Ideal posture is a stacking process where key points are aligned one over the other. The wall angel works by moving from a slouched posture to the opposite extreme by flattening out the curves in the spine. When one relaxes from the wall angel, posture is usually slightly improved. Doing the wall angel several times a day will start to change the body's default settings, so that eventually posture gets closer to the ideal.

Start by standing with your back against the wall with the feet 6 inches or more from the wall. Try to flatten your low back against the wall so that there is no space between the wall and your lower back muscles. Moving the feet farther from the wall and bending the knees will help flatten the back.

Once your back is flat, touch the back of your head against the wall. Keeping the low back flat and your head on the wall, bring your chin down by nodding the whole head slightly downward. Ideally, at this point you'll be looking straight ahead.

Next, raise your arms to 90 degrees at the shoulders with the palms facing the floor and the elbows at 90 degrees. The back of your upper arms should contact the wall. Keep your head on the wall and your back flat, and rotate the back of both arms up toward the wall. There may be a tendency for the low back to pull away from the wall. Rotate the arms up only as far as you can with good control.

The straight-arm wall angel and/or seated version may be substituted if you feel any problems in the shoulders. The Martian variation is an option if increased challenge is desired. Exercises are shown in Neck and Posture Exercises, p. 86–91.

WALL ANGEL

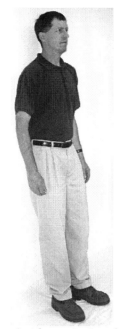

1. Stand with your back to the wall. Feet 6 inches or more from the wall.

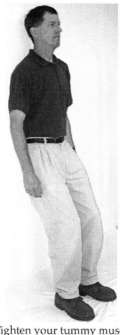

2. Tighten your tummy muscles to flatten your low back to the wall. Bend knees if needed to get back flat. KEEPING the back of your head on the wall, bring your chin down.

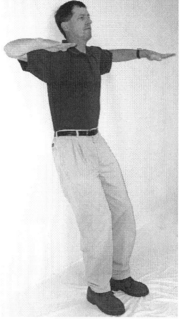

3. Put upper arms against the wall with palms facing down.

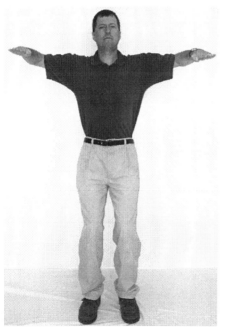

4. Keep back flat and your head on the wall with your chin down.

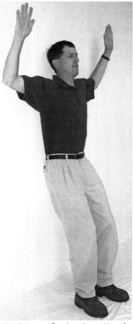

5. Move the backs of both arms to the wall.

Hold: 10-15 seconds.
Do 5-6 times per day.

Avoid Pain!

II
Advanced Hip Exercises

The preceding lying-down exercises prepare you to do the stand-up exercises. Once the lie-down exercises become easy, it's time to progress.

The hip muscles are designed to work when the foot is on the ground. All of the muscles in the buttock area are needed to control the center of gravity of the body in single leg standing, with every step you take. These muscles must keep the pelvis as level as possible. They must prevent the femur from angling and rotating inward. They also move you forward.

Walking can be broken down into several parts. The main components include heel strike, foot flat, and toe off for the leg touching the ground, and swing phase for the other leg. Walking differs from running in that both feet are in contact with the ground at the same time at some point. While running, only one foot at a time is in contact with the ground.

From heel strike to foot flat, the quadriceps and abductor muscles work to absorb shock and help stabilize the lower extremity and the pelvis. From foot flat to toe off, stabilization is still needed, and the gluteus maximus and other hip extensors kick in to provide propulsion to the next step.

Somewhat sloppy posture makes walking a controlled fall, with shock absorption by the anterior thigh muscles, including the quadriceps, hip flexors, iliotibial band, and spine. Propulsion then shifts down to the calf muscles, assisted by momentum of the opposite leg in the swing phase of walking. Often too much stabilization shifts up to the low back muscles or down to the inside portion of the thigh and knee.

Good closed chain functioning of the gluteal muscles is essential for unloading both the back and legs. Proper posture while walking or running allows the proper muscles to do the job nature intended.

REVERSE STEP LUNGE

The primary stand-up exercise for the gluteus maximus retraining is the reverse step lunge. Put a 3- to 6-inch-high platform against a door frame or facing a post. This platform can be an aerobic step, a block of wood, or magazines taped together. It must be stable.

Stand on the platform with one foot. Grab the door frame and touch it lightly with the top of your forehead. Place the other leg off to the side and extended behind you. Pull the toes up, and turn the leg inward. The bottom of this foot is parallel to the floor, and the heel is turned outward.

Holding the door frame firmly, perform a single leg squat by lowering the heel of the trailing leg towards the floor. The knee of your standing leg will bend, but do not let your shin move forward. Keep the standing shin stationary like a post in the ground. Most of the body weight will rest on the heel. Keep your forehead lightly touching the door frame throughout the movement. Monitor the shin visually and by the sense of weight remaining on the heel rather than moving to the ball of the foot.

This exercise is basically a single-leg squat with emphasis on moving the buttock back and reaching the trailing leg towards the floor. There is usually a tendency for the shin to move forward so the knee is over the toe. Try not to over-compensate by having your shin move backward, as this will usually over-engage the hamstring musculature. Keep your shin stationary!

Make sure the trailing leg stays off to one side and turned inward. The standing knee should be quiet during the entire exercise. Avoid popping or repetitive grinding in the knee. Making the motion shallower will usually relieve this problem.

If done correctly, the buttock muscles of the standing leg should do 90 percent of the work. Three sets of 5 repetitions once per day are usually sufficient for the first week. You may increase the repetitions as the exercise gets easier, but make sure you hit the target with each repetition of the exercise. The exercise is eventually done with only a light finger touch on the door frame for balance.

When repetitions become easy, holding a dumbbell weight against the hip of the trailing leg will increase the resistance of the exercise. Doing wall or door frame squats described later (pp. 49 and 37) may help to perfect the technique.

REVERSE STEP LUNGE

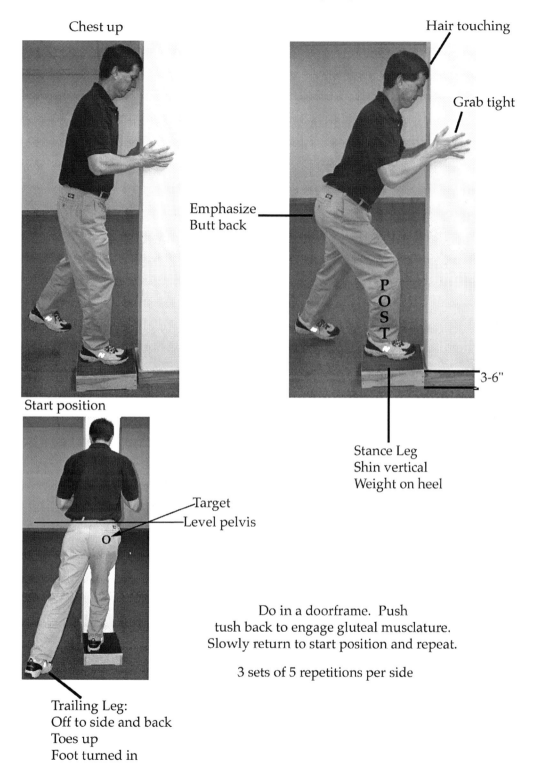

Chest up

Hair touching

Grab tight

Emphasize
Butt back

POST

3-6"

Start position

Stance Leg
Shin vertical
Weight on heel

Target
Level pelvis

O

Do in a doorframe. Push
tush back to engage gluteal musclature.
Slowly return to start position and repeat.

3 sets of 5 repetitions per side

Trailing Leg:
Off to side and back
Toes up
Foot turned in

Avoid Pain!

DOUBLE LEG DOOR FRAME SQUAT

An alternative to the reverse step lunge, the double leg door frame squat is usually somewhat easier, since both legs remain on the ground.

Place a dowel or broom/mop handle through a doorway flat on the floor 2 to 3 inches from the door frame. Position yourself so that either your toes or the balls of your feet are resting on the dowel. Your feet should be slightly wider than shoulder width and pointed straight forward. Grab the door frame and look down slightly. Touch your forehead lightly against the door frame.

Emphasize moving the buttock back, keeping the shins vertical. You need some degree of increased sway to your spine. If too much work is concentrated in the low back, tightening the abdominal musculature to a slight 12 o'clock or posterior tilt may help. Getting your thighs parallel to the floor is generally the maximum amount of movement, but stay within a comfortable range of motion.

If you do not feel the gluteal muscles are engaged after 3 to 4 repetitions, lower your hands to waist level before you start the squat. Clenching the buttock muscles at the bottom of the squat and before you come back up may help recruitment.

Avoid over-stressing the knees by monitoring sensations of strain, including noise in the knee. Three sets of 5 repetitions is usually a good starting point.

DOUBLE LEG DOOR FRAME SQUAT

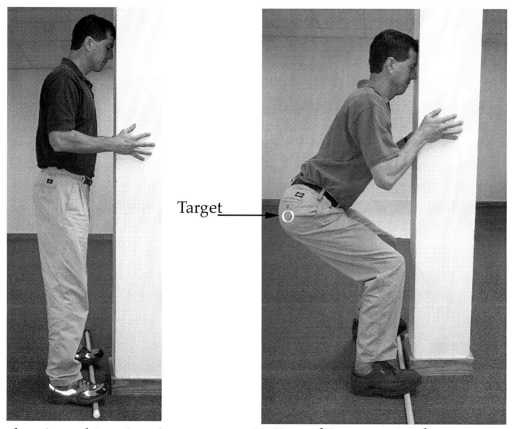

Target

1. Forehead touching doorframe or post. Dowel 2-3" from door. Grab tight.

2. Keep shin vertical. Chest up, butt back.

3 sets of 5 to start.

This can be used as an alternate to Reverse Step Lunge (p.34).

Avoid Pain!

Side Step Lunge/Hip Wobble with a Sit

This is a hip wobble with a sit motion aimed at the hip abductors. This exercise is a closed chain upgrade for the clam exercise. It is similar to the reverse step lunge in that you grab the door frame tightly, you stand on a block, your forehead touches the door frame, and the shin remains vertical.

Begin the exercise in a door frame, standing on a block with the inside edge of your foot close to the side of the block. Hang your free foot in mid-air and slightly ahead of the standing leg. Move your pelvis slightly back. Grab the door frame firmly, and keep your forehead touching the door frame.

Begin the motion by hiking the hip of the free leg (*i.e.* bring the pelvis towards the shoulder). Now "un-hike" or lower the pelvis down so the hip of the stance leg is pushed slightly back and slightly to the side. This is very much like the motion little kids do when they wiggle their backsides.

Sometimes it may be helpful to rest the fingers of the standing side arm behind the hipbone of the standing leg. As the opposite hip is hiked up, a hollow should develop in this area. As the hip is lowered, a bump should form. Once the wobble motion works, you should feel a slight fatigue in this area. Once this motion is perfected, add a slight sit motion by bending the knee at the down portion of the wobble. If you have painful or arthritic knees, do not add the knee bend. Just move back and forth from a hip hike to the un-hike.

Remember to keep the shin of the stance leg vertical and most of your body weight on the heel. This is similar to the reverse step lunge except that the hip is pushed slightly to the side as well as back. Move smoothly from the sit position back up to the hip-hike position.

Keeping the shin stationary is often a problem in the side step lunge. It will try to go forward when you are in the sit position, and hamstrings will try to pull it back when returning to the up position. Check it visually or have a partner lightly hold the shin just below the knee until you have reprogrammed yourself well enough to maintain good form. Keep the motion shallow in the beginning, and then increase the movement as the repetitions become easier. When correct repetitions of the exercise become easy, reduce the grip on the door frame.

Generally start the exercise with 3 sets of 5 repetitions. Increase the repetitions as you are able. When 15 or 20 repetitions are fairly easy, then begin adding the weight by holding a dumbbell weight against the hip of the free leg. If this exercise is too difficult, then try either the single leg door frame squat or the "ball on the wall" exercises that follow (pp. 40–43).

SIDE STEP LUNGE/HIP WOBBLE WITH A SIT

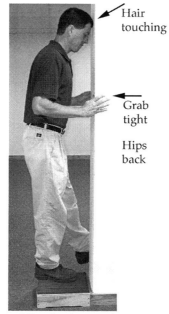

Hair touching

Grab tight

Hips back

1. Hips back, weight on heel.

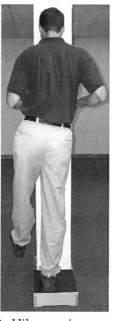

2. Hike or raise opposite hip upward.

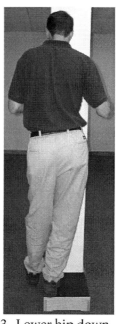

3. Lower hip down. Feel work behind hip bone on stance leg.

Do not let shoulders shift side to side or rotate.

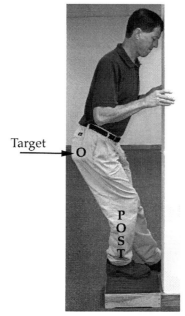

Target

O

P O S T

4. Lower further by bending knee,

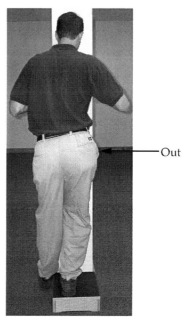

Out

5. and pushing hip out. Slowly return to hip hike position.

3 sets of 5 per side.

Avoid Pain!

SINGLE LEG DOOR FRAME SQUAT

A substitute for the closed chain activation of the hip abductors is the single leg door frame squat. Sometimes it is slightly easier than the side step lunge.

Position yourself in a door frame or against a post. If the door frame is narrow, position yourself at an angle. The top of your forehead lightly touches the door frame so that you are looking slightly downward. Tightly grab the door frame just above the level of your waist. Your lead foot touches the door frame, with the ball of the foot pulled up so that most of your body weight is on your heel. Imagine an egg under the ball of the foot. Your trailing leg is "on point" behind you and slightly to the side. Place a little pressure on these toes. This trailing leg remains planted as you move through the exercise. Think of it as a bicycle kick stand.

The motion of the exercise is similar to the reverse step lunge and the double leg door frame squat. Keep your chest up as you push your pelvis back. Keep your pelvis square and level. Level the pelvis by hiking the hip of the trailing leg. Do not over-compensate by moving the shoulders to the opposite side.

Try to keep the foot, knee, hip, and shoulder of the standing side in a line. Keep the motion fairly shallow when you start out. Maximum motion should not allow the thigh of the lead leg to go beyond 45 degrees from the vertical.

The work of this exercise should be felt behind the lead hipbone. If this exercise becomes too easy and you are doing it correctly, retry the side step lunge. Three sets of 5 repetitions is a good starting point.

SINGLE LEG DOOR FRAME SQUAT

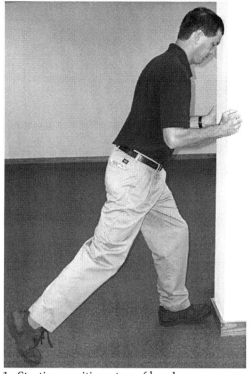

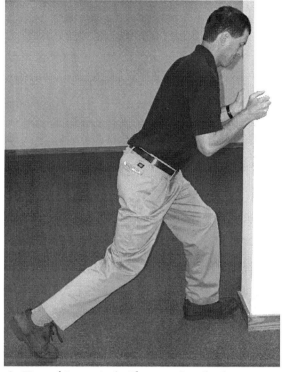

1. Starting position: top of head on doorframe, grab tight, egg under ball of foot, toe to door frame.

2. Keep shin vertical. Chest up, butt back. Keep pelvis square and level. Get tired behind lead hipbone.

3. Push tush back to engage muscle, then use muscle to return to the start position and repeat.

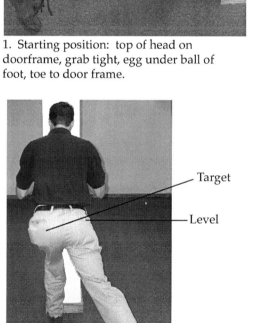

— Target

— Level

4. Keep planted. Light touch on toe.

3-5 lbs. of weight on toe of trailing leg.
3 sets of 5 per side.

Avoid Pain!

BALL ON THE WALL

A third way to recruit the hip abductor with a foot on the ground is to place a ball or a 6-inch diameter foam roller between your hip and a wall. Then you use the abductors on the outside leg to hike the pelvis to move the ball up and down on the wall.

If you are using a volleyball or basketball, stand with the ball held lightly against the wall with the side of your hip. Use just enough pressure to keep the ball in place. Ninety percent of your body weight should be on the outside leg, which can be slightly rotated inward. Rest your inside forearm against the wall for balance.

Roll the ball down the wall 5-6" by lowering the pelvis. The outside hip should push out. Roll the ball back up the wall by using the hip muscle of the standing leg. Fine-tune your positioning by turning your body in towards the wall and keeping your pelvis slightly pushed back. Try to localize the work to the area behind the hipbone. Two to three sets of 8 to 10 repetitions should be a good starting point for this exercise. Try the side step lunge (pp. 38–39) when this exercise becomes easy.

BALL ON THE WALL

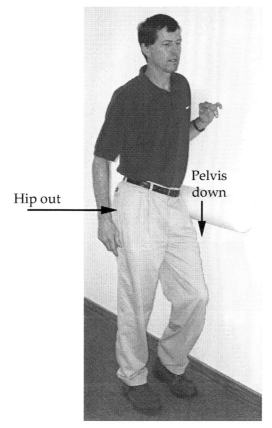

Hip out

Pelvis down

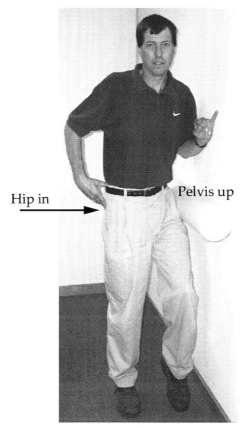

Hip in

Pelvis up

1. Use light pressure to hold ball or roller against wall. 90% of body weight on outside leg. Body is angled toward wall. Roll the ball down the wall 5-6". The outside hip should push out.

2. Now roll the ball back up the wall with the outside hip pushing the inside pelvis upward. Lower pelvis again to repeat the exercise. Get tired behind outside hip bone.

Do 2-3 sets of 8-10 per side.

Avoid Pain!

OLYMPIC SQUAT

This advanced hip exercise targets the gluteal muscles in your butt. Before attempting the Olympic Squat as a strengthening exercise, you should become proficient with the wall squat exercise (p. 48).

Once the wall squat has become easy, a natural progression would be to add weight to the exercise. Any squat or lift should be done as though there is a wall in front of you. Initially you can perform the wall squat with a bare bar.

Doing squats in a squat rack is recommended once you are adding significant amounts of weight. You can get good activation of the gluteal and paraspinal muscles by squatting to a level where the thighs are parallel to the floor.

When squatting, keep your body weight mostly on your heels to keep your shins as vertical as possible. This should prevent too much load from being directed toward the quadriceps and knees. Make sure that you can tap your feet throughout the squat motion to keep the shins in a reasonably vertical position.

Avoid letting the knees bow in or out. Knees should only bend like hinges, not universal joints. Your body weight should be distributed evenly so that each leg is carrying 50 percent throughout the squat.

Do your squats in 3 sets of 12 to 15 repetitions. Do the first set as a warm-up with 50 to 75 percent of your target weight. Do the next 2 sets with your target weight. A safe bet for your maximum target weight would be your ideal body weight.

Have an experienced helper or "spotter" available if you are inexperienced. Begin by removing the bar from the rack. Some people prefer backing up to the bar; others prefer to face it and duck under it to rest the bar on top of the shoulders. The bar should rest along the top part of the shoulder blades on top of the bony ridge. Add a pad or a towel around the bar for comfort. Grab the bar with your hands. Once the bar is resting comfortably on your shoulders, perform the squat as though you were doing your wall squat. Monitor knee and back positioning. Work should be felt through the buttock and back. If too much work is done through the quadriceps or low back, change your positioning as needed.

If you are unable to isolate the gluteal muscles correctly, continuing with the wall squat or single leg techniques (pp. 34–43) would be advisable.

OLYMPIC SQUAT

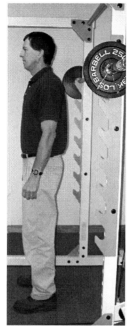

!. Squats with weights are done in a squat rack.

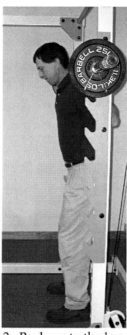

2. Back up to the bar. Put bar on shoulders.

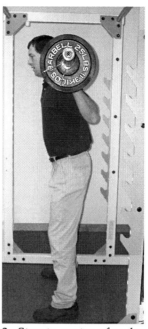

3. Step to center of rack.

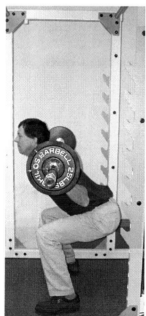

4. Squat down to thighs parallel to floor, shins vertical, chest up.

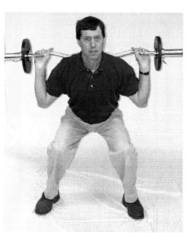

5. Keep knees neutral. Feet pointed straight forward.

Beginning Weight 25-45 lbs.
3 sets of 12-15 repetitions.

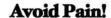

Avoid Pain!

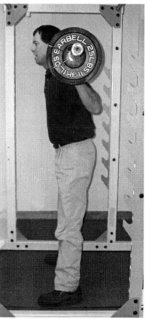

6. Back up to start position. Rise to start position and repeat.

III
Lower Extremity/Back Stretches

Stretching Guidelines

Stretching is an adjunct to a muscle re-education program. Stretching can decompress and restore full range of motion to joints. You can disinhibit muscles targeted for re-education.

Muscles that become tight and don't seem to loosen with regular stretching are muscles that are overly recruited on a regular basis. Stretching is not going to make a long-term change in the length of the muscle unless the overload is removed.

A muscle may become inhibited from functioning if its opposing partner muscle is tight. Tight hip flexors and other anterior thigh muscles may inhibit the gluteal muscles, causing problems in the back or legs. Tight pectorals (chest muscles) may inhibit scapular stabilizers, causing problems in the shoulder.

Stretching should feel good. Overly aggressive stretching may cause small injuries and soreness in the stretched muscle. This soreness results in more tightness, which is counterproductive to elongating the muscle. A gentle stretch can be held for a minimum of 15 seconds. A stretch can be held for 30 to 60 seconds if it produces the desired result of lengthening the restricted musculature.

Three to 4 repetitions of stretching with 15 to 30 seconds rest between stretches of the same muscle are generally sufficient for a session. If right and left sides are being stretched, one muscle gets a rest break while the opposite side stretches. Remember that overly aggressive stretching will actually slow the progress of elongation. Generally it is better to err on the side of a gentle stretch than stretching too hard.

Wall Squats

Wall squats can be thought of as a cousin to the wall angel exercise. Most people think it looks even sillier. This exercise works on making backward bending uniform through the lumbar and thoracic spine. It is also a good way to learn the Olympic squat technique professionals use to lift heavy weights safely. If done correctly, Olympic squats can be a good strengthening exercise for the gluteus maximus muscles (see p. 44). The wall squat will also help you learn good lifting technique.

Begin by facing the wall so your toes are touching the base molding. Point your feet straight forward slightly wider than shoulder width apart. Your hands can lightly touch the wall.

Begin the exercise by slowly sitting down and letting the pelvis push back and away from the wall. Keep the knees neutral and the feet flat on the floor. Squat only as far as balance and control will allow. You can hold the down position for 15 seconds as you would for the wall angel, or do repetitions. When returning to the start position, keep your nose (or cheek bone) lightly pressed against the wall.

Placing a dowel or broom handle across the ridge of the shoulder blades will usually increase backward bending through the thoracic spine. Doing this exercise with the feet only 2 inches apart tends to target more backward bending in the thoracic spine.

If pain or too much tightness is created in the low back, try a slight 12 o'clock or posterior tilt at the bottom of the squat to help neutralize the lumbar spine. Do not over-compensate and flatten the lumbar spine. Do the exercise within a comfortable range of motion. To increase the difficulty, move the feet closer together.

Other exercises that will improve backward bending include the door frame squat (pp. 36–41), door frame backward bending (p. 50), seated back extension (p. 74), attention (p. 80), and wall angel (p. 30).

WALL SQUATS

Stick

Target zone

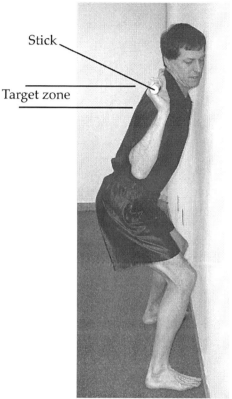

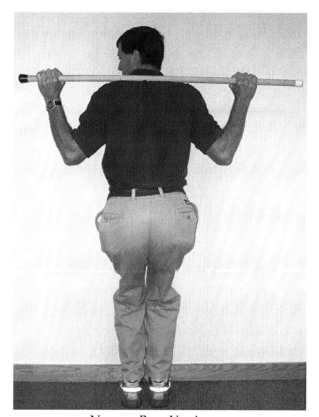

Wide Base Version   Narrow Base Version

Cheek and toes touch the wall.
Keep knees neutral and feet straight forward.
Keep the chest up as you push your butt back.
If needed do slight 12:00 tilt at the bottom of the squat.

Hold 15 seconds.
Can be used as an alternate to wall angel (p.30).

Avoid Pain!

49

DOOR FRAME BACKWARD BEND

This exercise works fairly well for improving and maintaining sacral motion. It can also be used as a generalized extension exercise. Since we tend to spend much of our time in a flexed position, the sacral motion may become restricted. This restriction does not allow the top of the sacrum to move forward to a neutral position when we stand. This loss of motion of the sacrum then transfers more work to the lumbar spine.

Place your fingertips over the depressions just inside the pelvic bones at the bottom of your back. Test if your positioning is correct by bending forward slightly; you should feel the depressions become shallower. Forward bending pushes the top of the sacrum back. Once your finger position is correct, back up to a door frame so that your heels, and thoracic spine touch the door frame.

Begin the exercise by letting your pelvis move away from the door frame. As your pelvis moves forward, you should feel the depressions deepen as the top of the sacrum moves into anterior nutation. Stay within a comfortable range of motion. Overall motion may be fairly small. Return to the start position and repeat this motion until you are comfortable with feeling the sacrum move. Moving too much may over-engage the low back.

You can add to this exercise by introducing a gentle sideways motion once your pelvis is moved away from the door frame. By gently letting your pelvis move to the left, you should feel the right depression become slightly deeper. By gently moving the pelvis to the right, the left dimple should become slightly deeper.

If your sacral motion is very restricted, it may be difficult to feel the depression. Manual therapy may be needed to restore the motion. Generally, the left sacroiliac joint is restricted in its forward motion more often than the right. The door frame backward bend can be used to gently nudge the top of the sacrum forward from a restricted position.

This exercise can be done several times a day. Hold 10 to 15 seconds in the restricted direction. Compare motion on the restricted side with the mobile side. If both sides are very restricted or if the side motions are painful, do just the first part of the exercise, and do not perform the left and right movements until more mobility is restored to the sacrum.

DOOR FRAME BACKWARD BEND

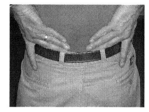

1. Finger tips in dimple area on back of pelvis.

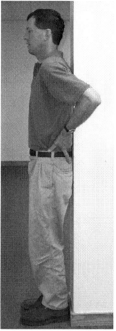

2. Back against doorframe. Heels against doorframe.

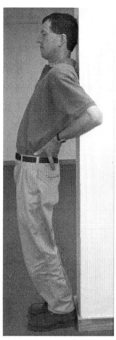

3. Let pelvis sway forward.

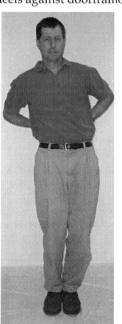

4. Then sway slightly to left, feel right dimple get deeper. Hold 10-15 seconds.

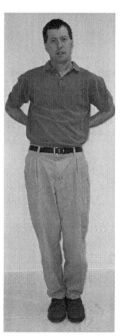

5. Then sway to right, feel left dimple get deeper. Hold 10-15 seconds

Repeat steps 4 & 5, 2-3 times each.

Avoid Pain!

KNEELING HIP FLEXOR STRETCH

Stretching the hip flexors may be needed to disinhibit the gluteal muscles, restore flexibility, and help correct posture. Tight hip flexors can cause anterior tilt of the pelvis and/or an increase in the lumbar lordosis or swayback. The work of the low back muscles increases to counterbalance the tension exerted by the hip flexors. If the hip flexors are tight, they may inhibit and weaken the function of the gluteal muscles.

There are several ways to stretch the hip flexors: kneeling, standing or lying. Start the by kneeling on one knee. Position the other leg with the hip and knee at 90 degrees each. The side that you kneel on will be the side that the stretch is applied to. Next tighten the abdominal muscles to flatten the low back with a strong 12 o'clock or posterior pelvic tilt. Try not to lean the upper body back. You might find it helpful to bend slightly forward from the waist. Use the hands to help with the pelvic tilt. The opposite hand is on the front of the pelvis, and the same side hand on the back of the pelvis. Tighten the buttock musculature on the stretch side. You should feel a stretch in the front of the hip on which you are kneeling. The opposite leg can now be used to pull your trunk forward. This should increase the amount of stretch.

Hold a gentle stretch for 15 to 20 seconds. Repeat 2 times. Generally a 15- to 20-second rest is required between stretches.

KNEELING HIP FLEXOR STRETCH

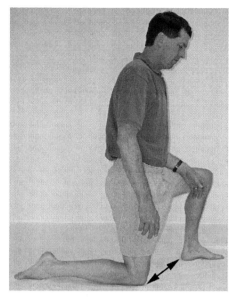

1. Have a wide base of support.

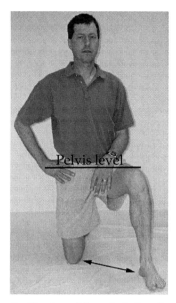

2. Begin with pelvis level.

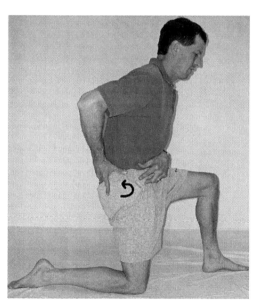

3. Strong 12:00 tilt. Use hands to help.
Tighten your butt.

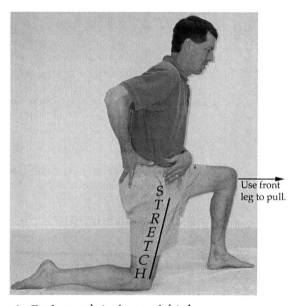

4. Feel stretch in front of thigh.
Cushion under knee if needed.
Hold 10-15 secs. per side. Do 2 per side.

Avoid Pain!

STANDING HIP FLEXOR AND QUADRICEPS STRETCH

Stretching of the hip flexors may be done from a standing position. This stretch requires some experimentation to find an object of a suitable height on which to rest the trailing leg. Usually a surface slightly higher than your knee works best.

Position a chair 4 to 5 feet in front of the object on which you are going to rest your trailing leg. Stand facing the chair, 12 to 18 inches away. Place the foot and ankle of the leg to be stretched on the trailing leg support. Tighten the abdominal musculature to flatten the low back and move the pelvis into a 12 o'clock or posterior tilt. Bend the standing leg to obtain a good stretch in the thigh of the trailing leg. Keep this knee close to the central line of the body, as it may be pulled to the side.

The stretch may be felt in the thigh anywhere between the knee and the front of the hip. As this area loosens up, you can increase the height of the trailing leg object or increase the length of your stance.

As with other stretches, hold for 15 seconds and rest 20 to 30 seconds between the stretches of the same muscle.

STANDING HIP FLEXOR AND QUADRICEPS STRETCH

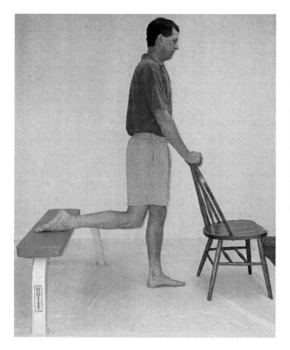

1. Place a kitchen chair in front of you for balance. Start with forefoot on a bench or chair behind you. Keep your upper body erect, tummy **tight** with low back **flat**. Position your stance leg far enough forward so the knee is comfortable.

2. Once positioned, bend the stance leg to the point of feeling a good stretch in the thigh of the leg behind you. Keep knee close to center line of body. Hold stretch for 15 seconds. Do 2-3 times per side, 2-3 times per day.

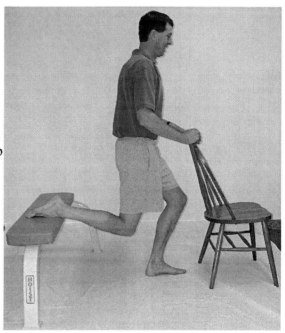

Avoid Pain!

SUPINE HIP FLEXOR STRETCH

If a more gentle stretch is needed for the hip flexor, a supine hip flexor stretch begins lying on a bed or couch so the side to be stretched is at the edge of the bed.

Lie on your bed with your hips 6 to 8 inches from the edge and your shoulders 12 to 18 inches from the edge. Bend your knees with your feet placed flat on the bed.

Bring your inside knee towards your chest and hold it with both hands. Let your outside leg ease off the edge of the bed towards the floor. Try to let this leg completely relax. Introducing some 12 o'clock or posterior tilt may increase the stretch. A partner can apply a light downward force above the outside knee if gravity does not provide enough stretch. Hold for 15 to 20 seconds. Repeat for 2 to 3 repetitions on the restricted side.

SUPINE HIP FLEXOR STRETCH

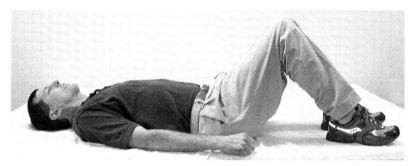

1. Lie on your bed with your hips 6 to 8 inches and your shoulders 12 to 18 inches from the edge.

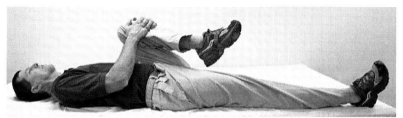

2. Bring your inside knee towards your chest.

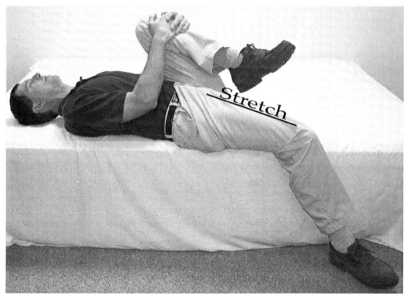

3. Ease the outside leg off of the bed.

2-3 stretches per muscle.
Hold 15-20 seconds each.

Avoid Pain!

HAMSTRING STRETCHES

The hamstring muscles run down the back of the thigh. The upper end attaches to the lower part of the pelvis and back of the thighbone. The lower end attaches below and to either side of the knee.

There are many ways to stretch hamstrings. Generally you want to maintain neutral or a slightly increased sway to the low back when doing either the seated or standing stretches to lessen the stress placed across the low back.

The door frame (or column) stretch may be used if you want your back completely unloaded or if you want a stretch that involves movement and stretch of the sciatic nerve. A belt placed over the ball of the foot can be used to apply extra force to the stretch. Often a pumping motion of the foot and ankle will help mobilize the sciatic nerve. Holding the ankle in a bent position and straightening and bending the knee will provide a similar effect. A static stretch for 10 to 15 seconds or 8 to 10 pumping motions is usually sufficient. This stretch can be repeated 2 to 3 times.

HAMSTRING STRETCHES

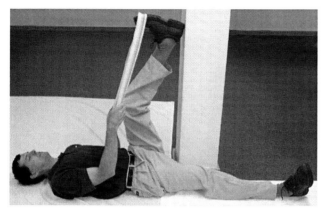

1. Doorframe (or column) stretch

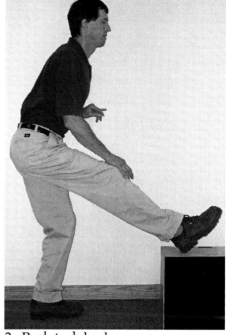

2. Push tush back.

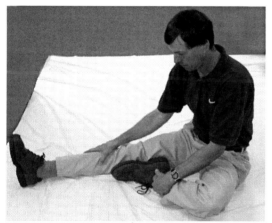

3. Lean forward from hips.

Some experimentation may be needed to find the stretch that best suits your abilities.

2-3 stretches per muscle.

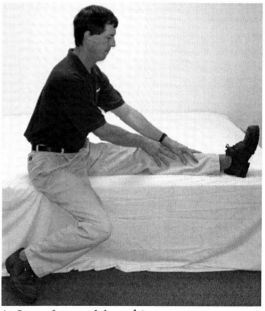

4. Lean forward from hips.

Avoid Pain!

QUADRIPED STRETCH FOR THE PIRIFORMIS

A more aggressive stretch for the piriformis and other small rotators of the hip may be accomplished in a quadriped position. It is essentially the upside down version of the piriformis stretch used as one of the basic 5 exercises for the low back (p. 16).

Begin the exercise on all fours. Position the leg to be stretched so the knee is under the center of the body, with the shin at a 45-degree angle to the long axis of the body. Slide the pelvis and the other leg back so that your body flattens down. Try to keep your pelvis level and square. It may be helpful to rotate the pelvis downward on the side of the trailing leg. To make the stretch more comfortable, you can rest on your elbows and forearms.

Roll to the side to get out of the stretch gently. As with other stretches, hold each stretch for about 15 seconds. Generally 3 repetitions are sufficient.

QUADRIPED STRETCH FOR THE PIRIFORMIS AND OTHER SMALL HIP ROTATORS

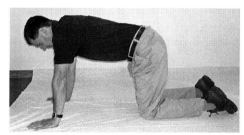

1. Start on hands and knees.

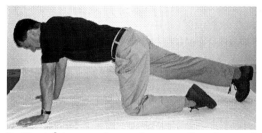

2. Straighten one leg and move other leg under the center of the body. The shin should be at a 45 degree angle to your spine.

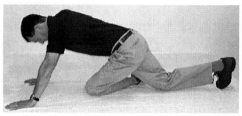

3. The foot of the leg under you should be under the opposite side of the pelvis.

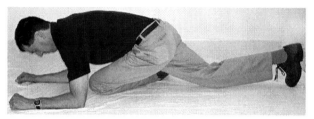

4. Now slide your pelvis and leg back so that your chest is over the knee that is under you.

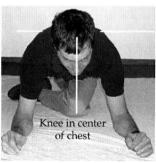

Keep pelvis level.

Knee in center of chest

Hold 15 seconds.
Do 3 per side.

Avoid Pain!

DEEP MASSAGE OF THE PIRIFORMIS MUSCULATURE

Occasionally the muscles deep in the hip are too tight, or even too knotted, to be affected by stretching. Piriformis syndrome may occur if the sciatic nerve becomes trapped within the muscles. This situation can simulate a pinched nerve. Deep massage is indicated if the area of the piriformis is very tender and if stretching with strengthening of the hip abductors and extensors does not resolve the problem.

The most effective application of massage is done with a stretch applied to the muscle. A massage therapist or "significant other" can be directed to massage the area with the subject in a side-lying position and the top leg pulled up towards the center of the chest. The massage therapist will find the tenderest area behind the hipbone of the top leg. Use pressure almost to the point of pain for 30 to 60 seconds. Small movements can be made in a circle, up and down, or side to side, with fingertips or an elbow.

If no one is available to help, then apply a self-massage using a tennis ball, or ball up a washcloth or sock. The ball is positioned beside the hipbone. The affected leg is pulled so that the knee comes toward the center of the chest, and then the hip is rolled onto the ball so that the ball is now under the piriformis muscles. Small oscillations will provide a deep massage. Adjust the size of the ball depending on the tenderness in the hip.

Massage can be applied to the piriformis muscles one to two times per day.

DEEP MASSAGE OF THE PIRIFORMIS MUSCULATURE

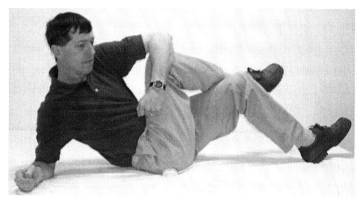

Position tennis ball or balled washcloth or sock under hip in tender area. Roll or move in small motions to deeply massage piriformis muscle for 30-60 seconds.

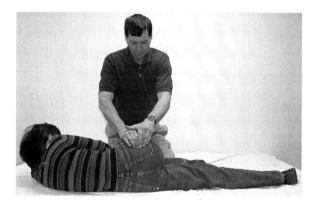 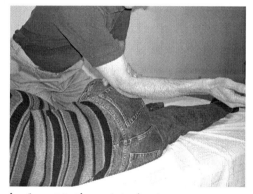

Have a significant other massage area. Push *almost* to the point of pain.

Do 1-2 times a day.

Avoid Pain!

STANDING CALF STRETCH

Occasionally it's necessary to stretch the muscles on the back of the leg between the knee and the ankle with a standing calf stretch.

Stand 12 to 18 inches from a wall. Your feet will be slightly wider than shoulder width apart. Place your hands on the wall at approximately chest height. Position the foot of the leg to be stretched 18 to 24 inches back from its original starting position. Turn this foot slightly inward and gently lock the knee straight. Keep the heel in contact with the floor. Bend the knee of the front leg slightly. Lean in towards the wall to increase the stretch in the calf. If more stretch is desired, move the trailing leg farther back.

A comfortable stretch should be held for at least 15 or 20 seconds. Again, 2 to 3 repetitions per side are optimal.

STANDING CALF STRETCH

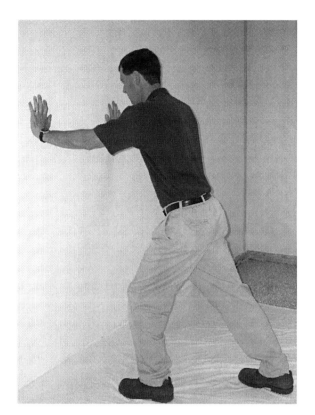 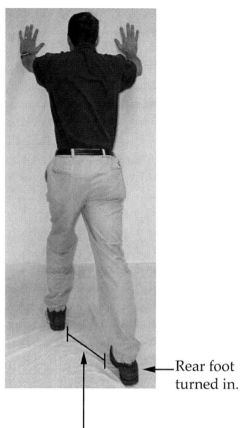

Rear foot turned in.

Shoulder width.

2-3 stretches per muscle.
Hold 15-20 seconds.

Avoid Pain!

BUTTERFLY STRETCH FOR THE HIP ADDUCTORS

Occasionally stretching of the hip adductors is helpful. These muscles run along the inside portion of the thighs.

Start a butterfly stretch by sitting on the floor with your pelvis and back against a wall. Position your legs so the soles of your feet are together. Lower your knees towards the floor. As you push the outsides of the thighs towards the floor, you should feel stretching along the insides of the thighs. You can increase the amount of stretch by pulling your feet closer to your groin area. More stretch can also be applied by grabbing your ankles and using your forearms and elbows to gently push your legs downward.

Hold the stretch for 15 to 20 seconds. Repeat 2 to 3 times.

BUTTERFLY STRETCH FOR THE HIP ADDUCTORS

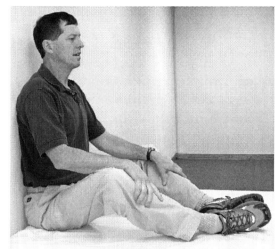

1. Sit with your back and pelvis against a wall.

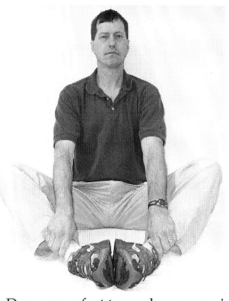

2. Draw your feet towards your groin.

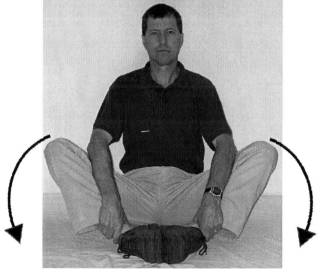

3. Use your forearms to push your legs down.

Hold 15-20 seconds.
Repeat 2-3 times.

Avoid Pain!

QUADRIPED LATISSIMUS DORSI STRETCH

The latissimus dorsi is a large muscle that runs from the low back to the armpit. This muscle can also be stretched from a standing or kneeling position.

The quadriped version of this stretch is accomplished by getting down on your hands and knees in front of a heavy object or door frame. Align one shoulder with the door frame one arm's length away. Grab the door frame with the hand of the arm that is not aligned with the door frame. Grab low to the floor with the thumb down. Now sit back, moving your buttocks towards your heels. As you sit back, try to increase the amount of "C" curve of the back. If the latissimus muscles are restricted, you will feel a stretch along the arm and down the side of the body.

Hold 15 seconds. Repeat this stretch 2 to 3 times on each side of the body.

QUADRIPED LATISSIMUS DORSI STRETCH

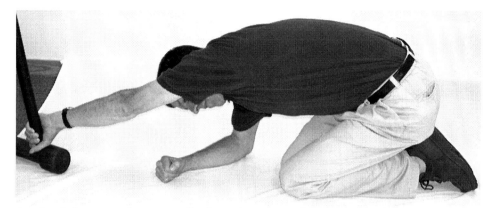

1. Grab heavy object with thumb pointed downward.

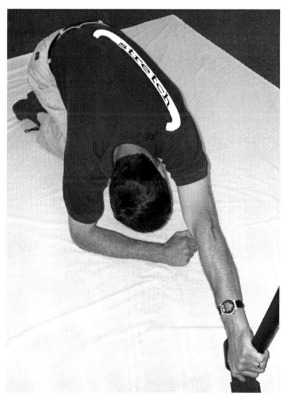

2. Sit buttock back towards heels to make a "C" curve in back. Feel stretch along "C".

Hold 15 seconds.
Do 3 per side.

Avoid Pain!

LATISSIMUS DORSI STRETCH WITH A CHAIR

This stretch may also help increase thoracic extension.

Start by kneeling in front of a bench or chair. You should be far enough from the bench so that when you lean forward, 5 to 6 inches of your upper arm will rest on the bench.

Rest your elbows on the bench so that your elbows are touching each other and bent at 90 degrees. Rest your forehead on your arms. Contract your abdominal muscles and move the pelvis into a 12 o'clock or posterior tilt. Then lower your chest towards the floor. This movement will be fairly small. You should feel stretching through the sides of the rib cage and central portion of the thoracic spine. You can increase the amount of stretch with a slight lowering movement of the hip towards the heels. Be careful not to cause pain in the shoulders.

Hold this stretch for 10 to 20 seconds. It can be repeated 2 to 3 times.

LATISSIMUS DORSI STRETCH WITH A CHAIR

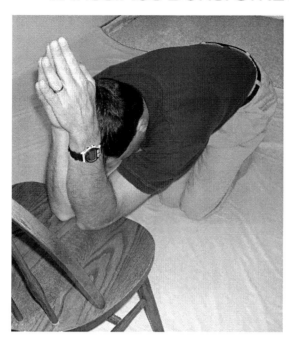

1. Kneel with elbows together on a chair. You should be far enough from the chair so that when you lean forward, five to six inches of your upper arm will rest on the bench.

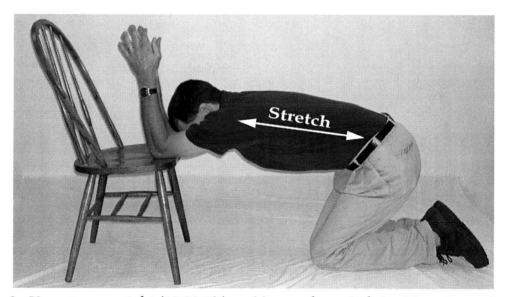

2. Keep tummy tight (12:00 tilt) and lower chest slightly. Move buttocks towards heels to increase the stretch.

Hold for 10-20 seconds.
Repeat 2-3 times.

Avoid Pain!

STANDING LATISSIMUS DORSI STRETCH

You can also stretch the latissimus dorsi from a standing position.

Stand with a wall 24 to 36 inches from your side. With your outside arm, reach over your head towards the wall. With the side bending motion, reach towards the wall and position both hands on the wall. If no stretch is felt, move your feet farther from the wall. You can also move the hips slightly forward or backwards to isolate the stretch to different fibers of the latissimus dorsi.

Repeat this stretch 2 to 3 times on each side. Each stretch can be held for a minimum of 15 seconds.

STANDING LATISSIMUS DORSI STRETCH

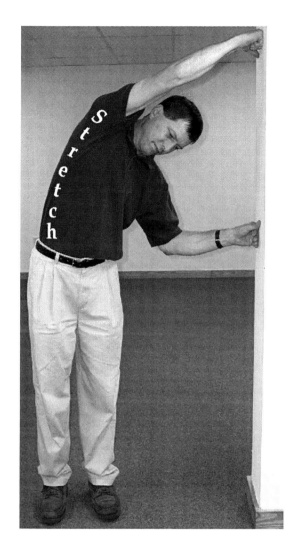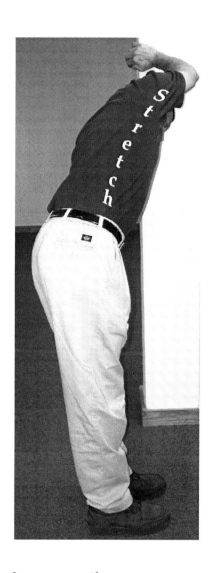

Position yourself to feel stretch along your rib cage.
Hold 15 sec. Do 2 to 3 times per side.

Avoid Pain!

SEATED BACK EXTENSION

This exercise can work to improve extension through the mid and lower thoracic spine.

On a firm straight-back chair, position a rolled-up towel in the restricted area of the upper back. Flex one leg so your foot rests on the edge of the chair. If this motion is restricted, then the foot can be placed on a stool or simply crossed over the other leg. Clasp your hands behind your neck and lean backwards over the towel roll. A slight contraction of the abdominal muscles may help isolate the movement to the thoracic spine.

Alternate legs with each stretch. Hold each stretch for 10 to 15 seconds. Repeat 2 to 3 times on each side.

SEATED BACK EXTENSION

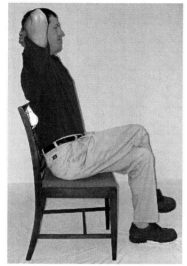
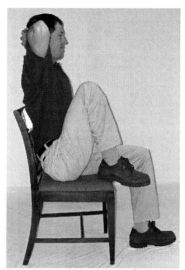
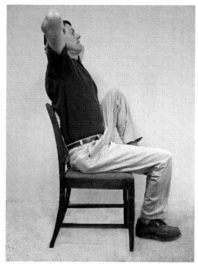

1. Roll a small towel so that it makes a firm roll 2-3 inches thick. Sit with back against chair, roll aligned at the restricted level.

2. Place a foot up on chair (or crossed).

3. Place hands behind neck and lean backward until you feel a stretch.

Hold 10-15 seconds.
Relax, switch legs and repeat.
2-3 repetitions per side, 2-3 times a day

Avoid Pain!

IV
NECK AND POSTURE EXERCISES

The following exercises balance muscular control and restore mobility in both the neck and upper back areas, which are key elements for postural control.

Imbalance in the cervical region involves overuse of the scalene, levator scapulae, upper cervical extensors, and trapezius muscles, which then become tight, and underuse of the deep neck flexors and thoracic extensors, which then become weak. Poor backward bending mobility in the thoracic spine can cause forward head posture. To level the head, the scalenes and upper cervical extensors are overused.

The scalenes, in addition to providing support for the head and neck, assist in breathing. They help lift the chest when extra lung volume is needed. Many people tend to breathe in the upper chest rather than with the diaphragm. The upper-chest breathing pattern can be reinforced by sedentary and/or stressful lifestyles. An upper-chest breathing pattern adds work to the scalene musculature, which may increase the tendency toward poor posture. It may also cause the upper rib cage to remain in an elevated position.

The scalenes and upper rib cage are intimately associated with the nerve and blood supply to the arms. The brachial plexus starts out from nerve roots exiting the spinal column. These nerves pass through the scalene musculature, over the first and second ribs, under the collarbone, and under the pectoral muscles to get to the arm. If there is dysfunction in any of these areas, you can get symptoms in the arm that include weakness, pain, tingling, burning, or numbness.

The muscles in the back of the neck include the levator scapula, upper trapezius, and many small suboccipital muscles. With forward head posture, these muscles may become overused. Tightness and soreness can result.

The levator scapulae and trapezius musculature attach to the head and neck, and to the scapulae or shoulder blades. They stabilize the shoulder blade, and help control the head and neck. If too much of their work is devoted to the head and neck, tightness and pain can result.

If posture is poor, significant mechanical dysfunction may occur in the suboccipital joints and in the upper cervical spine, aggravating and/or causing problems with headache and the temporal mandibular joints. The temporal mandibular joints are where the jawbone attaches to the face, in front of the ear canals on either side of your face.

Retraining the function of the deep neck flexors must be done in conjunction with improving function in the thoracic spine. Since most of our daily activities involve some degree of flexion or bending forward of the thoracic spine, we tend to lose the ability to extend this part of the spine back to a neutral position. Using a towel roll or foam roller will help passively restore motion. The attention and wall angel exercises will help restore muscular control. Occasionally the pelvic clock is needed if poor control of the abdominal muscles is found. Stretching of the scalenes and/or levators may be helpful. The following exercises can be done in any order, and are generally done twice a day. The wall angel can be done several times during the day for micro breaks.

The other exercises in this section are adjunct exercises for neck, shoulder, and upper back problems, and each one can be used on an as-needed basis.

PLAY DEAD

Retraining the deep neck flexors is paramount for reprogramming correct posture. Play dead is one of the better exercises for isolated retraining of these muscles.

Why is it called "play dead?" Imagine playing a game with a 6-year-old. You are playing dead. You think that the child is near your feet. If the child sees you tuck your head, lift and look, then you are out of the game. So a very subtle tuck, lift, and set down are required to keep playing!

Start by lying on your back on the floor. Your knees can be bent or straight. Fold a bath towel widthwise so it is 5 to 6 inches wide, and place it under the upper back so the top edge of the towel runs across the top of the shoulders. Look straight at the ceiling.

Tuck the chin by nodding the head downward toward the toes. While maintaining this tuck, lift the back of the scalp no more than one-eighth of an inch from the floor. Hold this position for only one to two seconds, and then lower slowly.

Imagine an axle or rod placed through the ears; this nodding motion causes rotation around the axle. The slight lift is a continuation of the rolling motion.

Once you do the first tuck, lift, and relax sequence to the center, then turn the head slightly to one side and repeat the tuck, lift, and relax sequence. Turn the head only far enough so that one eye is looking straight up. Repeat the same sequence with the head turned slightly in the other direction. This exercise is generally done in sets of 5.

Remove the towel from under the shoulders if it is too uncomfortable, or if it makes the exercise too difficult. If needed, place a folded towel under the head. This may be required if your posture is extremely compromised with severe forward head posture.

The exercise can be further modified by eliminating the lift portion. Just gently tuck the chin and hold this position for 4 to 5 seconds. Turn slightly, re-tuck and hold, and then repeat in the opposite direction. When the tuck portion of the exercise becomes easy and comfortable, gradually add the lift. Introduce the towel under the shoulders if the lying flat version becomes easy.

PLAY DEAD

Lie on back, folded towel under shoulders.

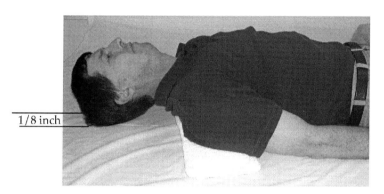

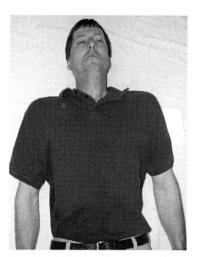

1/8 inch

1. Tuck chin, lift head LESS THAN 1/8 of an inch. Hold 1-2 seconds. Relax slowly.

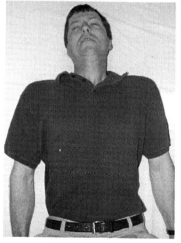

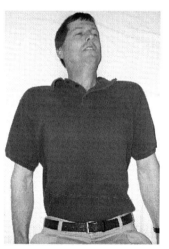

2. Turn very slightly to the right, tuck, lift, relax.

3. Turn very slightly to the left, tuck, lift, relax.

Repeat sequence 5 times/twice a day.

Avoid Pain!

ATTENTION: SUPINE VERSION

In this exercise, you lie on your back at attention. This easy exercise may serve as a good starting point if the neck or low back is irritable. It may also work well if the thoracic spine is very rigid or the muscles poorly recruited.

Lie flat on your back. Your knees can be bent or straight. If needed, place a folded towel under your head. Tuck the chin with the same nodding motion in play dead, then gently press the back of the head down against the floor. Gently squeeze the shoulder blades together towards the center of the spine. This squeeze should cause the breastbone to gently rise toward the ceiling. Try not to arch the low back. Focus the tension between the shoulder blades. Hold this position for 3 to 5 seconds, and then relax for 10 to 15 seconds before repeating. In the beginning, 5 to 6 repetitions will be sufficient.

As it becomes easier and your repetitions increase to 10 to 12, you may try to progress to the prone version.

Attention: Supine Version

Flat on back

Tuck chin

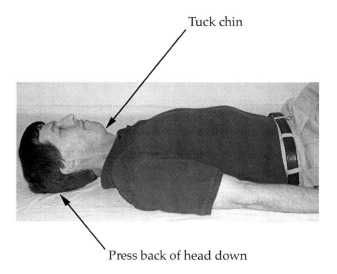

Press back of head down

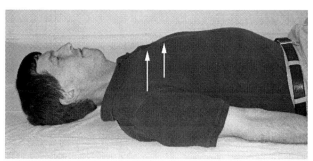

Pinch shoulder blades together to push breast bone upward.
Keep low back relaxed.

Hold 3-5 seconds.
Focus the tension between the shoulder blades.
Start with 5-6 repetitions and work up to 10 to 12 over two weeks time.
Twice per day.

Avoid Pain!

ATTENTION: PRONE VERSION

The attention exercise is designed to isolate the function of the thoracic spine extensors and, to some degree, the scapular stabilizers. The scapular stabilizers on the back of the body help pull the shoulder blades towards the center of the back. There are two basic versions of the exercise. One version is done in a prone position (on the stomach), and the other is done in a supine position (on the back, p. 80). If the prone version proves either painful or just too difficult to coordinate, try the supine version.

For the prone attention exercise, you need one to two pillows, a rolled-up hand towel, and a "lump." This lump can be an ace wrap, balled washcloth, or a folded sock.

The pillow goes under the stomach area, generally no higher than the bottom of the rib cage. The lump is placed under the upper part of the breastbone below your throat. Your forehead rests on the rolled towel. Your arms will be at your sides.

Once positioned, begin by pressing your breastbone down against the lump. Without lifting from the lump, retract your shoulder blades by pulling them to the center of the back and slightly downward towards the low back. Now lift your head very slightly while keeping the chin tucked, and then press down into the lump again.

At this point, you are lying face down at "attention." You should feel work or tension between the shoulder blades. Hold this position for 3 to 5 seconds and repeat 5 to 6 times, with 5 to 10 second rests between repetitions.

The exercise may be modified by eliminating the head lift portion. Adding an extra pillow under the abdominal area and/or repositioning the pillow may also help. If this version still proves too difficult, then the supine version may be easier.

ATTENTION: PRONE VERSION

Face down with pillow under tummy and head on rolled towel. Balled washcloth or sock for "lump" under breast bone.

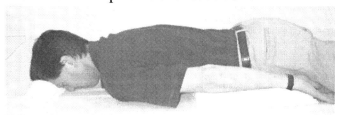

1. Press chest down to "lump".

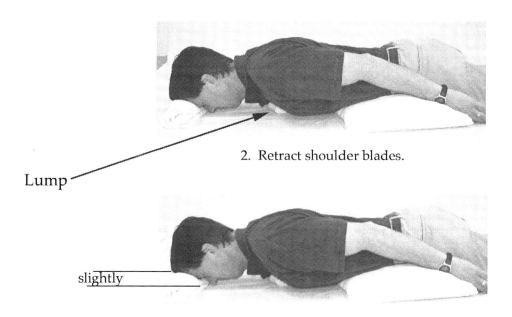

Lump

2. Retract shoulder blades.

slightly

3. Lift head slightly with chin tucked.

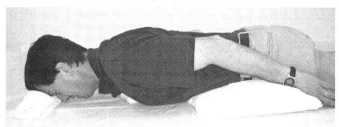

4. PRESS AGAIN!!!
Hold 3-5 seconds. DON'T LOOK UP!
Focus the tension between the shoulder blades.
Start with 5-6 repetitions and work up to 10 to 12 over two weeks time.
Do twice per day.

Avoid Pain!

TOWEL ROLL

The attention exercises work on increasing muscular control in the thoracic spine. The towel roll works on increasing mobility. The towel roll plus the 12 o'clock tilt and raising the arms over your head, can also improve shoulder mobility and provide a stretch for the latissimus dorsi muscles.

Do the towel roll exercise on the floor. An exercise mat may be used. You will need one or two hand towels and a bath towel or small pillow for supporting your head. Roll two hand towels together widthwise. Place them on the floor and position yourself on the towel roll so that it runs from the base of your neck down to the bottom of your rib cage, centered in your back. Your head should be supported in a comfortable position with your pillow or folded bath towels. Your legs can be bent, straight, or propped on a chair. Place your arms wherever they are comfortable.

Generally, lie on the towel roll for 10 minutes. Do the arm stretch every 2 minutes.

Before raising the arms, tighten the tummy slightly and perform a 12 o'clock or posterior tilt. Slightly tuck the chin, and then raise the arms over your head as far as they will comfortably go while keeping the elbows straight. If discomfort occurs in the top of the shoulders, move the arms either closer together or farther apart. Hold a stick in your hands if you are dealing with a shoulder problem. Hold this stretch position for 15 seconds and repeat every 2 minutes while on the towel roll.

When your thoracic spine begins to loosen up, you may increase the size of the towel roll up to 3 towels. When 3 towels no longer provide a good push, you might consider the foam roller exercises described later in this book (p. 161).

TOWEL ROLL

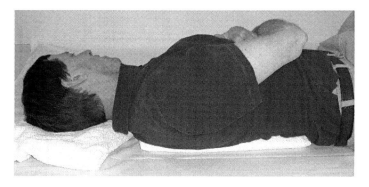

Lie on 1-2 rolled up hand towels placed lengthwise under the spine. Start the towel at the base of the neck.   Head supported.

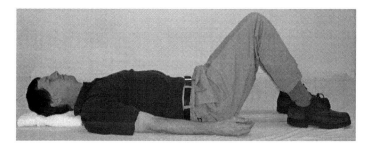

Lie on towel for total of 10 minutes.

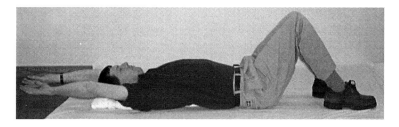

Every 2 minutes raise the arms over head and hold for 15 seconds. (Hint: tighten the tummy and tuck the chin when raising arms.)

Avoid Pain!

WALL ANGEL AND ITS VARIATIONS

The wall angel combines all of the neck exercises into one stand-up version. When standing up, you need the parts to stack up, and the muscles control you once you are there. Lie-down exercises can improve muscle function and mobility, but the change in postural programming must be done in the vertical mode.

If coordinating the angel is too difficult, there are several variations. See Variations p. 91 and Seated Wall Angel p. 89. Excluding the arms portion can modify the wall angel. If your low back and/or head will not touch the wall, then get them as close as you can without undue discomfort.

This exercise does not have to be executed perfectly to be beneficial. If you feel work or stretch with this exercise, it is probably taking you in the right direction. If the standard wall angel proves too difficult in the stand-up mode, try the seated wall angel.

Start by standing with your back against the wall with the feet 6 inches or more from the wall. Try to flatten your low back against the wall so that there is no space between the wall and your lower back muscles. Moving the feet farther from the wall and bending the knees will help flatten the back.

Once your back is flat, touch the back of your head against the wall. Keeping the low back flat and keeping your head on the wall, bring your chin down by nodding the whole head slightly downward. Ideally, at this point you should be looking straight ahead.

Next, raise your arms to 90 degrees at the shoulders with the palms facing the floor and the elbows at 90 degrees. The back of your upper arms should contact the wall. Keep the head on the wall and the back flat, and then rotate the back of both arms up toward the wall. There may be a tendency for the low back to be pulled away from the wall. Rotate the arms up only as far as you can with good control. Hold this position for 10–15 seconds. You may do one or two wall angels 5 to 6 times throughout the day.

STANDARD WALL ANGEL

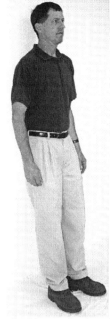 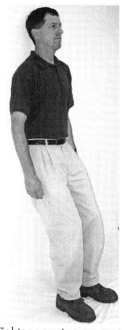 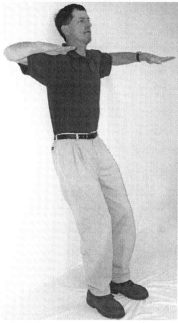

1. Stand with your back to the wall. Feet 6 inches or more from the wall.

2. Tighten your tummy muscles to flatten your low back to the wall. Bend knees if needed to get back flat. KEEPING the back of your head on the wall, bring your chin down.

3. Put upper arms against the wall with palms facing down.

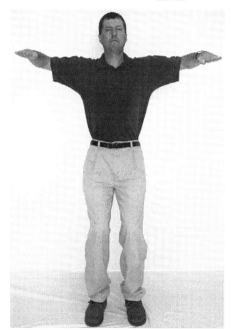 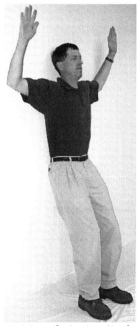

4. Keep back flat and your head on the wall with your chin down.

5. Move the backs of both arms to the wall.

Hold: 10-15 seconds.
Do 5-6 times per day.

Avoid Pain!

SEATED WALL ANGEL

The seated version of the wall angel may work well if you have substantial difficulty flattening your low back against the wall.

Using a low stool or sturdy chair with its side pushed against the wall, sit with your back to the wall and flatten your lower back against the wall. Try to touch the back of your head against the wall while keeping your low back flat and your chin down. If you find it too difficult to touch the wall with either the low back or the head, then come as close as comfortable. Hold this position for 10 to 15 seconds and repeat it 5 to 6 times during the day.

If you can touch your head to the wall and keep your low back flat, position your upper arms against the wall so that a straight line is formed from one elbow, through your shoulders and to the other elbow. Bend the elbows at 90 degrees with the palms and forearms parallel to the floor.

Keeping the back flat and the chin down, slowly rotate your arms so the forearms and hands go up towards the wall behind you. Go as far as comfort and control will allow. The low back must stay as close to the wall as possible. A sensation of work or stretch may be felt through the upper back, neck, or across the shoulders. Hold this position for 10 to 15 seconds and repeat five to six times during the day. Progress to the standing version if this becomes easy.

Use a straight elbow version if you experience pain or other problems in the shoulders.

SEATED WALL ANGEL

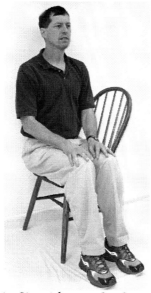

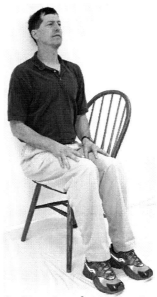

1. Sit with your back to the wall. Tighten your tummy muscles to flatten your low back to the wall.

2. Keeping the back of your head on the wall, bring your chin down.

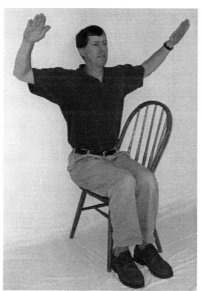

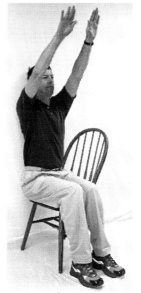

3. Start with your palms facing the floor. Move the backs of both arms towards the wall.

4. Straight arm version.

Hold 10-15 seconds.
Do 5-6 times per day.

Avoid Pain!

MORE WALL ANGEL VARIATIONS

The straight elbow version of the wall angel may be used if shoulder problems prohibit the rotation or positioning used in the standard wall angel. If raising the arms still causes shoulder pain, the exercise can be further modified by grabbing a cane or stick and raising it so that one arm can help the other. The exercise is still executed with the low back flat against the wall and the head against the wall with the chin tucked down.

Another wall angel technique might be called the "Martian variation." Start with the low back flat and the chin tucked as before. Raise your arms in front of you with the elbows fully bent and the elbows as close together as possible. Your palms can be turned towards the ceiling and the backs of your fingers will touch the wall beside your head.

Keeping the fingers on the wall and your elbows close together, push your hands toward the ceiling, causing the elbows to straighten. Stretch may be felt between the shoulder blades or along the sides of the chest.

Hold a comfortable stretch for 15 to 20 seconds. Take the arms as high as comfortable. Avoid the tendency for the elbows to push out to the sides. A single arm version can be employed if the double arm version is too difficult. Use your free hand to help push the arm upward. If the arms are very weak, a family member may assist by pushing the arms upward.

Hold the positions for 15 to 20 seconds and repeat 2 to 3 times. This exercise can be done several times during the day.

MORE WALL ANGEL VARIATIONS
Variation #1, Straight Elbow

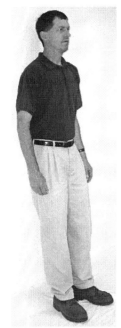 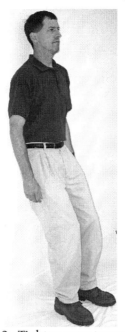 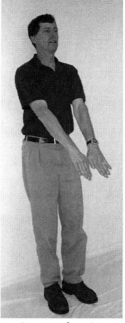 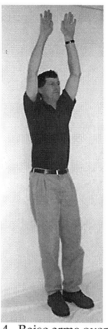

1. Stand with your back to the wall. Feet 6 inches or more from the wall.

2. Tighten your tummy muscles to flatten your low back to the wall. Bend knees if needed to get back flat. KEEPING the back of your head on the wall, bring your chin down.

3. Start with palms facing the floor.

4. Raise arms over head towards wall.

Variation #2, Martian
Steps 1, 2 are the same as above

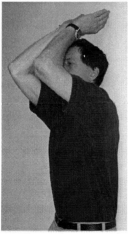 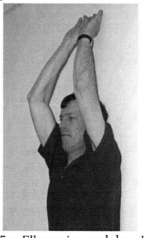 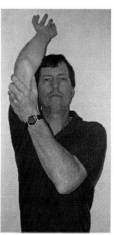

4. Elbows bent, touch fingers to wall just overhead.

5a. Elbows in, push hands up the wall.

Hold 10-15 seconds.
Do 5-6 times a day.

5b. If both arms are difficult, do single arm.

Avoid Pain!

CUEING FOR POSTURE

For retraining posture, I like the foot tap, look ahead exercise.

To determine if this exercise will help you, try to tap your feet alternately. Do you have to shift your shift your weight back onto your heels, or throw your shoulders back, or rock your body side to side? If so, this exercise may help with posture correction.

Start by looking at your shoestrings or at the top of your socks. For most people, this shifts the pelvis back so you can now tap your feet. Keeping the pelvis back, lift the chest and head so you are looking straight ahead. Do not let the pelvis come forward. This may entail keeping a little tension in the abdominal muscles. Now shrug the shoulders up and down and then forward and back two to three times. Can you still tap your feet? Initially this may feel awkward, but with practice, default setting will change, and correct posture will feel more natural. Repeat this exercise several times throughout the day.

CUEING FOR POSTURE: "LOOK DOWN, LOOK AHEAD"

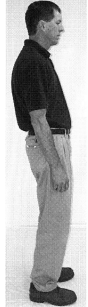
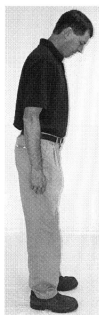
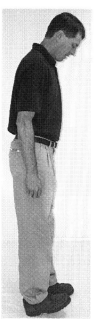
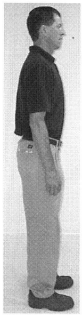

1. Poor posture.

2. To correct poor posture, look down at shoe strings or top of socks.

3. Tap feet. Note that pelvis is back.

4. Look ahead but don't let pelvis come forward.

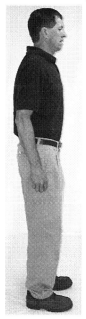
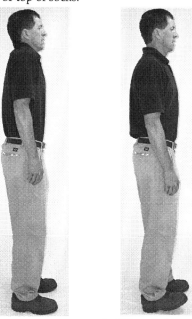

5. Roll shoulders in a circle, 2-3 times.

6. Relax slightly. Make sure you can tap your feet without shifting your body position.

Repeat every 30 minutes when standing.

Avoid Pain!

ARM STRETCH

Tightness in the chest and upper arm is probably the result of compromised posture. Once tight, these restrictions may further protract the shoulders. Tightness in the pectoral muscle may inhibit the use of posterior scapular stabilizers. These include the rhomboids and lower and middle trapezius muscles. This results in overuse of the upper trapezius and rotator cuff muscles. This exercise will stretch your chest and upper arm muscles.

Begin the stretch standing beside a wall. The little toe of your inside leg should be touching the base molding with the foot at a 45 degree angle to the wall. The outside foot should be parallel to the inside one, shoulder width apart. Your chest should be at 45 degrees to the wall.

Position your inside arm with the palm on the wall, elbow straight, so that it is 45 degrees down from the horizontal. If you start with the arm at your side and raise it up the wall, you will stop when it's approximately half way up. Your shoulder should remain in contact with the wall with your outside hand flat on the wall in front of your chest. Stand up straight, don't let your head rest on the wall, but do face forward.

At this point, you may feel some stretch in the front of the arm that is on the wall. To increase the stretch, gently rotate the body to increase the angle of the body in relation to the wall by pushing with the hand that's in front of the chest. If you can rotate your body so that it is 90 degrees to the wall and without feeling a stretch, reposition the chest back to 45 degrees and raise the arm three to four inches. Push again to rotate the body away from the wall. If you can get your arm to horizontal and your body to 90 degrees, then you probably do not need this stretch.

If pain is felt in the shoulder, you can lower the arm below 45 degrees. The arm can be rotated so that the thumb and forefinger are against the wall. If this does not make the exercise comfortable, try introducing the stretch by grabbing a doorknob and turning your body so that stretch is applied. When this can be done comfortably, try the wall again.

Hold each stretch for 10 to 15 seconds. Repeat 2 to 3 times per side. This exercise can be done several times during the day.

ARM STRETCH

Push to rotate body.

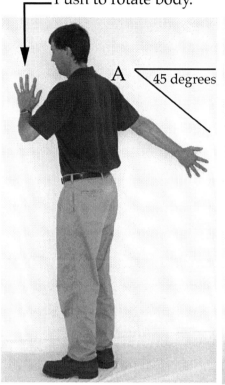

A 45 degrees

1 Month

1. Starting position:
Little toe against baseboard.
Feet: 45 degrees to wall.
Chest: 45 degrees to wall.
Arm: 45 degrees from horizontal.

2. Push to rotate body to increase stretch in front of arm that is on the wall

Hints: Keep shoulder "A" in contact with wall
Hold 10-15 seconds
Do 2-3 side
Do 2+ times per day

Avoid Pain!

SELF STRETCH FOR MEDIAN NERVE DISTRIBUTION
(AFTER DAVID BUTLER)

The nerves that service our arms start at the mid and lower portion of the neck as nerve roots. The nerve roots join together to pass through the scalene muscles, then over the first and second ribs. From there they pass under the collarbone and chest muscles. The median nerve begins at the border of the chest muscle at the upper arm. From there, it travels along inside the upper arm to the front of the elbow. It then dives into the muscles of the front of the forearm and travels through the carpal tunnel to anchor into and innervate the thumb, index, and middle finger.

Restrictions in movement of the median nerve through this course can cause numbness and tingling which are symptoms of nerve root impingement, and can be a contributor to carpal tunnel syndrome.

The median nerve stretch will help move the nerve through its tortuous course, and restore the movement needed for optimal functioning.

Begin by positioning your arm like a waiter carrying a tray. Keep your palm facing the ceiling and your fingers pointing away from your body. Keep your shoulder down by placing the opposite hand on top of the shoulder and exerting a downward pressure. Extend your arm by straightening your elbow directly to the side. Keep your hand at the same height as your shoulder with the wrist fully extended. Straighten your arm to the point of feeling a stretch in the forearm or front of the elbow.

Looking in a mirror may help maintain ideal positioning. Keep the shoulder down and the wrist fully extended. The arm should be moved directly out to the side of your body. A stretch can be held for 10 or 15 seconds. A pumping motion may be employed in which you straighten the arm to the limit of stretch, then relax it slightly and repeat the straightening. Do for 8 to 10 repetitions. Leaning the head away from the arm being stretched will increase the amount of pull. This exercise can be repeated several times during the day.

SELF STRETCH FOR MEDIAN NERVE DISTRIBUTION

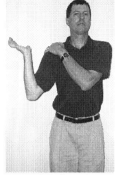
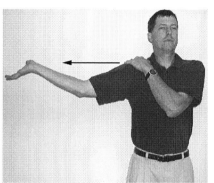
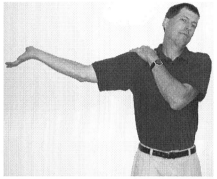

1. Hold shoulder down wrist fully extended.

2. Straighten elbow. Keep shoulder down and wrist extended.

3. Increase stretch by leaning head to opposite side.

Variation

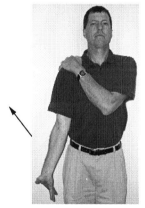
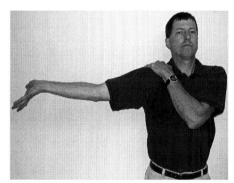

Keep elbow straight and wrist extended. Raise arm to engage comfortable stretch.

Hold 10-15 seconds or bend and straighten elbow or wrist several times.

Avoid Pain!

UPPER CERVICAL SOFT TISSUE RELEASE

Occasionally deep soft tissue work will be beneficial in loosening the suboccipital muscles located along the back of the neck just under the base of the skull. Problems in this area include restrictions in motion, tightness, and tenderness. Impingement on the suboccipital nerves may contribute to headaches and/or restriction in motion in the cervical spine. This exercise can be done either from a sitting or a side lying position.

The side lying technique is probably the most effective, but good results can be obtained either standing or sitting. If one side is more restricted, then lie on the opposite side so that the sore side is up. Do not use a pillow unless absolutely necessary. Position your head so that the area above your eye is resting on the surface of whatever you are lying on. Your top arm will rest along your side, and the hand of the bottom arm will be used to massage the suboccipital area. The spots that will benefit most from the massage are usually the most tender. Massaging for the purpose of loosening is most effective when a slight stretch is applied. Knead the restricted area for 30 to 60 seconds per square inch. Apply pressure that is sufficiently firm to work on the underlying tissue. This pressure may be almost to the point of pain.

This technique can be repeated several times a day on any area that you find that is restricted.

UPPER CERVICAL SOFT TISSUE RELEASE

Sidelying Version

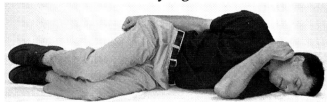

1. Lie on your side with top arm resting along top side of body.

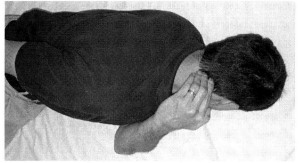

2. Rotate slightly downward to obtain best stretch. Massage on any areas that feel tight or tender.

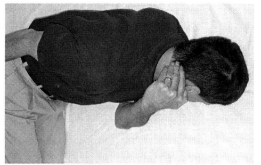

3. Use opposite hand to reach behind neck to provide deep soft isssue massage.

Sit/Stand Version

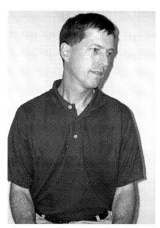

1. Rotate the head slightly to one side.

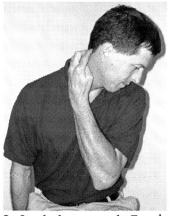

2. Look downward. Reach around with the opposite hand to provide deep massage to the upper neck.

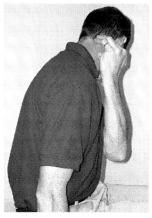

3. Adjust rotation to get the best stretch.

Press hard enough to provide a deep massage
but not so hard as to elicit pain.
Work on restricted areas for 30-60 seconds. 2-3 times a day.

Avoid Pain!

UPPER TRAPEZIUS/LEVATOR SCAPULAE STRETCHING

The upper trapezius attaches to the back of the neck and base of the skull, and drops down to attach along the top of the shoulder blade. The levator scapulae attach along the back of the vertebrae of the neck and to the top, inside corner of the shoulder blade.

Stretching these muscles can be done from either a standing or sitting position. Start by sitting in a chair. If you are stretching the right side, your right arm will be at your side. Turn your head 45 degrees to the left, tip your head slightly to the left, and now look down toward the left side of your pelvis. Adjust the rotation and side bending to find the stretch that will be best felt along the back of your neck into the top of your shoulder blade.

Grabbing the seat of the chair with the right arm so that the right shoulder does not elevate can increase the stretch. You can also rest the left hand on top of your head and let just the weight of your arm increase the amount of stretch. Reverse the directions to stretch the other side.

Each stretch should be held for 15 to 20 seconds and can be repeated 2 to 3 times per side. Stretching can be done up to several times a day.

UPPER TRAPEZIUS/LEVATOR SCAPULAE STRETCHING

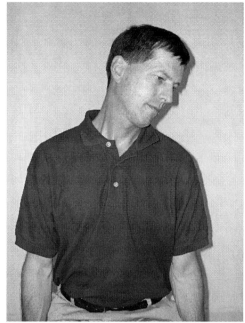

1. Tip your head to the side. Rotate slightly to the same side.

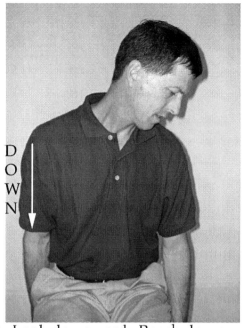

2. Look downward. Reach downward with the opposite arm.

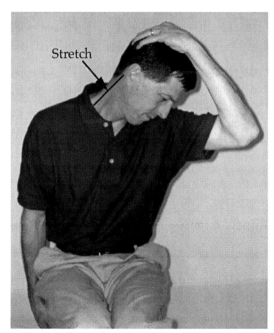

3. Place the other hand on your head to provide extra stretch.

Hold 15-20 seconds. Do 2 to 3 per side.

Avoid Pain!

SCALENE STRETCHING

The scalenes are in the front of the neck on either side of the throat. One end attaches to the sides of the vertebrae, and the other end attaches to the first and second ribs behind the collarbone.

Stretching of the scalene muscles can be done from either a standing or sitting position. The right scalene is stretched by placing the base of the left thumb in the soft area above the right collarbone at the base of the neck. The rest of the palm cups over the collarbone so that the inside border of the little finger is on the underside of the collarbone. Apply a downward pressure, not over the collarbone but over the portion of the rib cage above and below it. This downward pressure stabilizes the bottom attachment of the scalenes.

With the bottom of the scalenes stabilized, tip the head slightly to the left and rotate it slightly to the right. Let the head tip back as you would if you were looking up with only your right eye. The back of the head will be aiming downward towards the back of the left shoulder. This should provide a stretch from the jawbone down to the collarbone on the right side. Adjusting rotation and tipping your head will fine-tune the stretch. Lifting the jaw towards the ceiling may also facilitate stretching.

Each stretch should be held for 15 to 20 seconds and can be repeated 2 to 3 times per side. Stretching can be done once or up to several times a day.

SCALENE STRETCHING

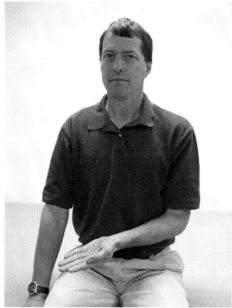

1. Align your thumb with your index finger.

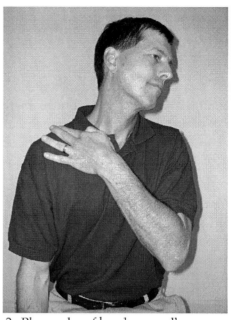

2. Place palm of hand over collar bone so that thumb is above the bone.

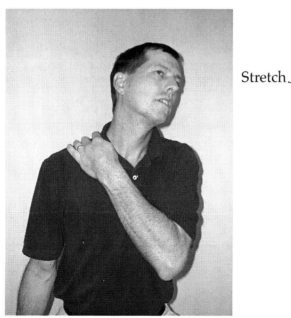

3. Press downward with hand. Tip your to the opposite side, and rotate slightly to the same side.

Stretch

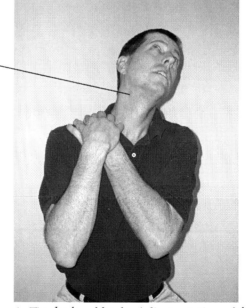

4. Tip the head back. Adjust rotation of the head and neck to get best stretch. Use other hand to add support.

Hold 15-20 seconds. Do 2 to 3 per side.

Avoid Pain!

DIAPHRAGM BREATHING

A diaphragm-breathing pattern has many advantages over an upper-chest-breathing pattern. Musicians and singers tend to be diaphragm breathers, which is a much more efficient pattern than using accessory muscles to lift the upper chest.

Compromised postural habits and poor aerobic capacity may lead to a change from a diaphragm-breathing pattern to an upper-chest-breathing pattern. When one takes in a deep breath and the lower rib cage and abdominal area expand outward, that is diaphragm breathing. There is a slight straightening of the spine as the diaphragm draws air into the lower portion of the lungs.

In an upper-chest pattern, a deep breath causes mostly lifting of the upper chest with very little expansion of the lower rib cage. With this pattern, the scalenes, because of their attachment to the upper ribs, provide much of the lift for upper chest breathing. This pattern contributes to overuse and subsequent tightening of the scalene musculature.

Retraining of the breathing pattern can be done by monitoring movement of the chest and/or the lower rib cage with the hands. You can also monitor visually by doing the exercise in front of a mirror.

Begin by placing the hands lightly along the lower rib cage so that the middle fingers line up at the bottom of the sternum or breastbone. Now take in a slow, deep breath by making the lower rib cage push outward. When the breath is relaxed, the ribs and abdominal area will naturally return to their starting point. Repeat this several times. You may have to inhibit the tendency to move the upper chest consciously.

Another technique would involve inhibiting the upper chest movement by placing the hands on the upper chest and consciously restricting the movement in this area with inhalation. Sometimes one hand on the upper chest and the other across the upper abdominal area will give better feedback. Any of the above hand placements can be used while watching in a mirror.

With a little practice, retraining of the breathing pattern will help reduce overuse of the scalenes. If this exercise proves challenging, repeating it several times a day for 4 to 5 repetitions would be helpful.

DIAPHRAGM BREATHING

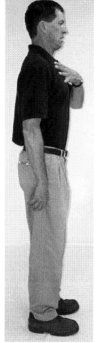

1. In a stress pattern of breathing, the upper chest lifts with inhalation.

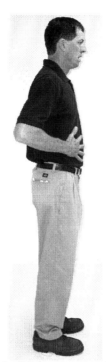

2. With an optimal breathing pattern, the lower ribs move out with inhalation.

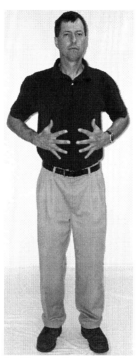

3. Correct breathing by monitoring movement of chest and ribs with hands.

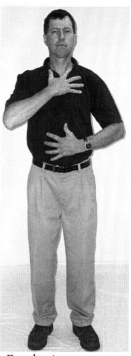

4. Emphasize movement of lower ribs while lessening the movement of the upper chest.

Monitor several times during the day.

Avoid Pain!

DOOR FRAME PULL DOWN

This exercise is designed to activate the back extensors and scapular stabilizers. You will need a four-foot piece of latex band or bicycle inner tube.

Tie a knot in the center of the latex band and place it over the top of a door; close the door to hold the knot. Grab the band at eye level with the palms facing forward, the little fingers on top, and the thumbs pointing downward. Bend your elbows so the arms almost form a circle.

The movement of the exercise opens the circle. The elbows remain bent at a constant angle and the shoulder blades squeeze back and down toward the center of the back. You should feel tension between the shoulder blades. Slowly relax to the starting position. Repeat for 2 sets of 8 to 10 repetitions. Adjust the arms up or down to get the best work out of the exercise.

DOOR FRAME PULL DOWN

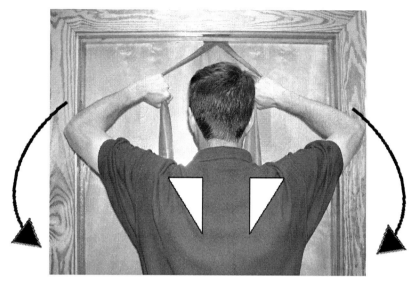

1. Grab band with thumbs down. Start motion by squeezing shoulder blades.

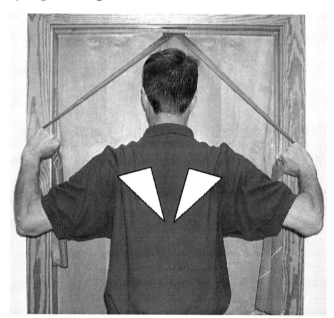

2. Let arms move in a circular motion. Try not to let elbows bend.

Do 2 sets of 8-10 repetitions.
Rest 30 seconds between sets.

Avoid Pain!

UPPER THORACIC SEGMENTAL RETRAINING

Restrictions in backward bending motion of the upper thoracic spine tend to pitch the head forward and contribute to a "hump back" appearance. The foam roller and rolled towel techniques will help loosen the area (p. 161). The following technique will help you regain active control.

Sit in a straight-back chair. Place your index fingertip in the space between two of the largest big bumps at the base of the neck. Nodding the head slightly will help in identifying the correct position. Now place the fingers of the opposite hand on top of the first fingers and bring your forearms forward to hold under the jawbone or around the sides of the face. The elbows should point straight forward. Position the lower trunk in a 12 o'clock or posterior pelvic tilt.

From this position, the arms, head, and neck should move as a solid unit with most of the motion occurring at the segment under your fingers. The motion is small. Move the arms (head and neck) slightly downward to feel the space open. Now move the arms upward. Hold for 1 to 2 seconds, and then relax. Now lift the elbows slightly to the right, hold, and relax. Lift slightly to the left, hold, and relax. Position the head and neck back at the center, and then reposition the fingers down into the next interspace. Repeat the above exercise. If a segment is extremely restricted, you may repeat the lift/relax sequence several times. You can repeat this technique as far down as your fingers can reach. If significant relief is provided, this exercise may be done several times per day.

UPPER THORACIC SEGMENTAL RETRAINING

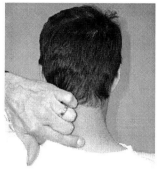 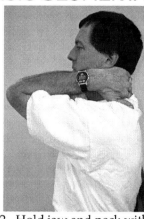

1. Start at interspace where good movement is identified.

2. Hold jaw and neck with forearms. Hold the spine and pelvis in a 12:00 or posterior tilt.

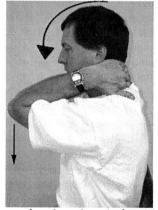 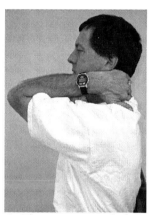

3. Arms, head, and neck should move as unit. Move down slightly. Feel the interspace open.

4. Then move up slightly. Feel the interspace close. Back to neutral.

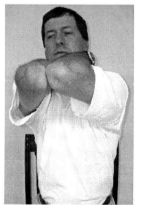 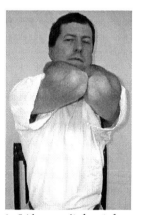

5. Then lift at a slight left angle.

6. Lift at a slight right angle.

Repeat lifts to center, right and left 4 times at each level that you can reach.
Do this exercise 4-5 times per day

Avoid Pain!

V
Advanced Abdominal Exercises

The following exercises strengthen the abdominal muscles and train the muscles as part of a guy-wire system. During upright activities, the muscles that surround the trunk from the rib cage to the pelvis function mainly as a guy-wire system. The only time the abdominal muscles function as a sit-up or crunch muscle is when you get out of bed in the morning. Once you are up, you need these muscles to balance the tension of the back muscles.

Sit-ups and crunches also have a tendency to increase flexion or bending forward of the thoracic spine. Most activities in our modern society will do this for us; therefore, exercises that promote flexion should be minimized.

The following three exercises can be done to strengthen the abdominal muscles in a way that does not increase flexion of the thoracic spine.

SUPINE HEEL TOUCHDOWN

Lie on your back on the floor with your knees bent and your feet flat. Your hands can help with motion control by placing them on the abdominal muscles, or under the back, or by grabbing the pelvic bone.

First, perform a strong 12 o'clock or posterior tilt. The tummy muscles should be pulled flat and tight, and the low back should be "glued" to the floor. With the posterior tilt established, bring first one thigh and then the other to 90 degrees with the knees relaxed. Retighten the 12 o'clock tilt. Now slowly lower one leg to lightly touch the heel to the floor before returning it to the 90-degree starting position. Repeat the process on the other side. Concentrate on keeping your tummy tight, your back flat, and your pelvic bones rotated into the 12 o'clock direction. Alternate sides and complete 2 to 3 sets of 8 to 10 repetitions.

If abdominal control is poor, take the heel only halfway towards the floor before returning it to the 90-degree position. As the exercise gets easier, extend the leg farther out. Always make sure the back is flat and the abdominal muscles tight.

SUPINE HEEL TOUCHDOWN

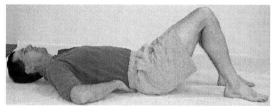 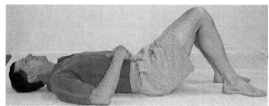

1. Lie on back with knees bent. Place fingers under small of back or on abdomen.

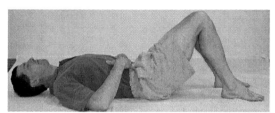

2. Do a strong 12:00 tilt to flatten low back.

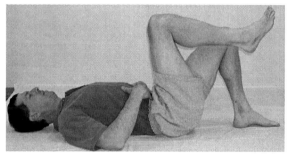 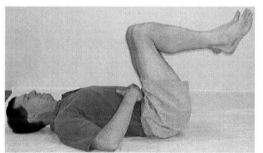

3. Bring one knee to 90 degrees.

4. Bring other knee up. Retighten the 12:00 tilt and tuck the chin.

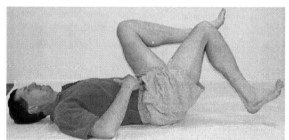 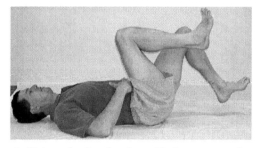

5. Slowly lower one heel towards the floor. Do not let the distance between rib cage and pelvis increase. Lightly touch the heel.

6. Bring the leg back to 90 degrees and repeat on the other side. Alternate sides.

Do 2-3 sets of 8-10 repetitions.

Avoid Pain!

ABDOMINAL BRIDGE OR PLANK

With correct positioning, the bridge can provide you with a good isometric contraction of the abdominal muscles.

Begin by resting face down on your elbows and forearms. Your upper arms will be at 90 degrees to your body. Straighten your body so your hips and knees are straight and you are resting on the tips of your toes. Tighten the abdominal muscles so the pelvis is moved into a slight 12 o'clock or posterior tilt. Hold this position for 30 to 45 seconds. You can repeat it 3 to 4 times as part of your abdominal workout.

ABDOMINAL BRIDGE OR PLANK

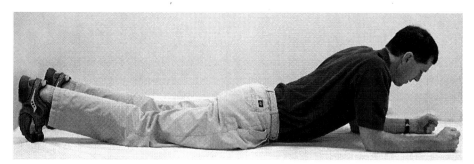

1. Rest face down on elbows and forearms.

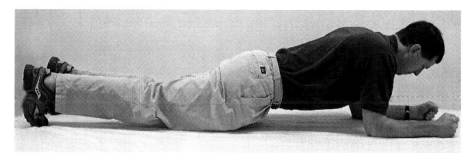

2. Straighten knees to prop on elbows, forearms, and toes.

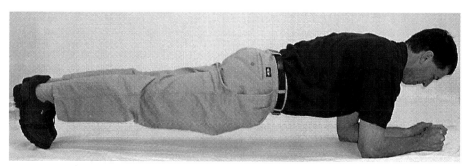

3. Align the shoulders, hips, ears, and ankles. Keep tummy tight and tucked.

Hold 30-45 seconds.
Do 3-4 repetitions.

Avoid Pain!

ADVANCED ABDOMINALS: CHAIR EXERCISE

Another option for abdominal strengthening is done with an office chair or rolling stool. It works similarly to the rolling devices advertised on TV.

Begin by kneeling in front of an office chair. Place your elbows and forearms on the seat of the chair. Stabilize the upper arms at an approximate 90-degree angle to the body. Let the chair roll forward by gently pushing with the hips and knees. Keep the abdominal muscles tight so the spine does not sag downward. Keep the head aligned with the shoulders.

Roll forward as far as good control will allow, then return to the starting position. Keep the tummy tight throughout the entire motion.

Rolling at a slight angle will help recruit the oblique abdominals. A sequence of rolling straight, then back to neutral, slightly to the left (back to neutral), and then slightly to the right (back to neutral) would be considered one repetition. Repeat 8 to 10 repetitions in 2 to 3 sets.

ADVANCED ABDOMINALS: CHAIR EXERCISE

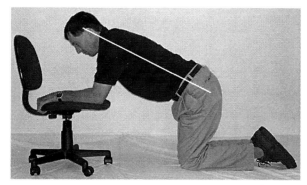

1. Starting position.

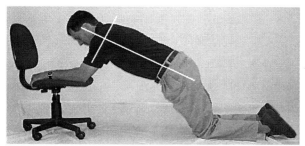

2. Push chair outward. Keep shoulders and arms stationary. Use abdominal muscles for control of out and back motion. Stay within range of control.

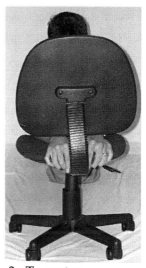

3. To center.

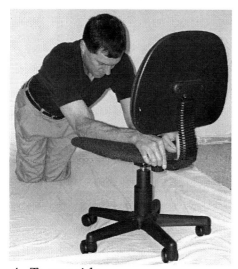

4. To one side.

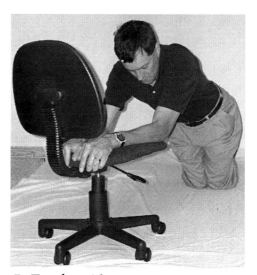

5. To other side.

2-3 sets of 8-10 repetitions.
30 seconds rest between sets

Avoid Pain!

VI
Upper Body Exercises

Posture and overall function can be improved with correct execution of upper body exercises. The neck and posture exercises discussed earlier can be made almost unnecessary if a good upper body-strengthening program is followed on a regular basis.

For most people, a free-weight exercise program works best for several reasons. It is portable and can be done at home or in a gym. The exercises facilitate control of postural muscles rather than letting a machine provide that control. The techniques can be modified to suit a given body type or functional restrictions. You can also design a free-weight program to target a specific area or to train for a specific activity.

General training and conditioning are usually done with a program that emphasizes high repetitions and lower weights. High repetitions generally mean 12 to 15 repetitions. These exercises are generally done in 2 sets of 12 to 15 repetitions with a 30 to 60 second rest between sets. Each exercise is done with sufficient weight so that the targeted muscle group is fatigued by the end of the set, and good form is maintained.

Good form means maintaining good posture and/or alignment while exercising to target a muscle group. Avoid pain! Each movement of the exercise should be slow and controlled, taking at least 2 to 3 seconds per direction of each movement.

If an exercise causes pain, try to modify the exercise by decreasing the movement or decreasing the weight. If pain persists with a specific exercise, try another exercise that targets the same muscle group. A 10- to 15-minute warmup period is recommended before starting an exercise session. This can include walking, biking, or light jogging.

The upper body free-weight exercises are divided into three groups: chest, back, and shoulders. An exercise session would consist of 1 or 2 exercises from each group. Free-weight exercises can be done every other day or 3 days a week. Try to vary the exercises and the order in which each group is done with each session. An exercise session can also include advanced abdominal exercise as well as closed chain hip exercises. Generalized quadriceps, hamstring, and calf exercises can be included for the legs, and biceps and triceps exercises for arms.

A high repetition, low weight workout will generally increase strength, tone, and control, but not increase muscle bulk. Working with a personal trainer may help with correct execution of the exercises as well as with guiding you in a general fitness program.

TYPICAL 3-DAY WORKOUT SCHEDULE

DAY 1	DAY 2	DAY 3
Warm-up	Warm-up	Warm-up
Reverse and side step lunges	Olympic style squats	Reverse and side step lunges
Chest: Bench press and bench fly	Lateral shoulder: upright row and incline lateral raises	Back: Bent over row and frontal pull down
Lateral shoulder: Door frame lateral raises and upright rows	Chest: Incline dumbbell press and bench fly	Lateral shoulder: Door frame lateral raises and frontal raises
Back: Single arm row and incline reverse fly	Back: Seated reverse fly and seated row	Chest: Incline dumbbell press and bench fly
Abdominals: Supine heel touchdown and abdominal bridge	Abdominals: Chair exercise and supine heel touch downs	Abdominals: Supine heel touchdowns and bridges
Optional: Incline bicep curls and supine elbow extension	Optional: Quadriceps, hamstrings, and calf work	Optional: Extremity work

UPPER BODY EXERCISES FOR THE BACK

SEATED REVERSE FLY

Scapular retractors include rhomboids and lower and middle trapezius muscles. These muscles pull the shoulder blades towards the center of the back. The seated reverse fly exercise targets these as well as the spinal extensors of the thoracic spine. Very often, this exercise is started without any weight. As the repetitions and sets get easier, add weight.

Sit on a low bench or in a chair with knees and feet together. The knees are partially extended to form a 45-degree angle. There are two ways to arrive at correct trunk positioning for this exercise. The first is bending forward so that the chest is resting on the knees with your arms hanging straight down. Lift your upper body keeping the abdomen as close to the thighs as possible. Try to achieve alignment of the ears, shoulders, and hips. Look toward your toes. This positioning can also be achieved by leaning forward from the hips so the abdomen is close to the thighs and the chest is lifted upward.

Once in the correct position, raise the arms by squeezing your shoulder blades. Let the shoulder blades pull the arms up to horizontal. The arms should now be straight out from your sides with the palms facing the floor. You should be able to see your hands with your peripheral vision. Elbows should be almost straight. We call this the "piper cub" configuration (like the little straight wing airplane). If the muscles are very weak, there is a tendency for the arms to angle back in a "delta wing" configuration. This positioning is easier but not as effective at targeting the muscles. Let the arms return to their starting position and repeat the exercise.

If positioning or pain is a problem, the next exercise, the incline reverse fly may be a better choice (p. 126).

SEATED REVERSE FLY

Target: Back

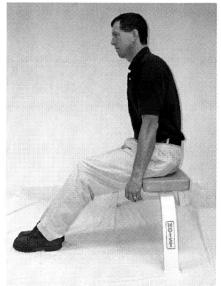

1. Knees bent at 45 degrees.

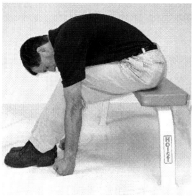

2. Rest chest on knees.

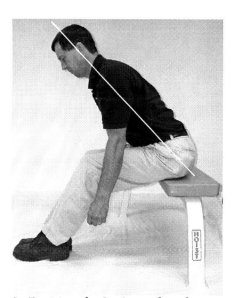

3. Position the body so that there would be a straight line from the ears, shoulders to the hips. Look at your toes.

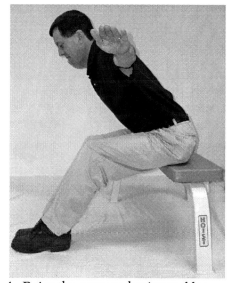

4. Raise the arms to horizontal by squeezing the shoulder blades together. Maintain "piper cub" configuration, not "delta wing". Lower arms slowly and repeat arm raise.

2 sets of 12-15 repetitions.
Beginning weight 0 lbs.

Avoid Pain!

INCLINE REVERSE FLY

The incline reverse fly is usually easier than the seated reverse fly, but it requires a weight bench that will incline. This exercise is generally started with 2 to 5 pounds of weight.

An adjustable incline bench should be raised to a 45-degree angle. Lie face down on the bench with your chin or forehead down. The hips should be at an approximate 90-degree angle to your body. Your arms hang down with your elbows straight but not locked.

Raise your arms by squeezing your shoulder blades together and letting the shoulder blades pull your arms to horizontal. Palms should be facing the floor, and the arms should be straight out from your body with the elbows still not locked. You should see your hands with your peripheral vision. Lower your arms slowly and repeat.

INCLINE REVERSE FLY

Target: Back

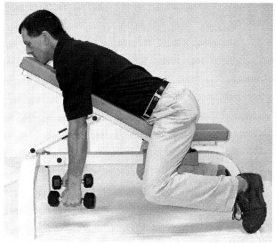 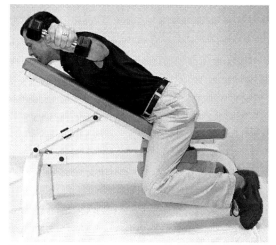

1. Incline bench at approximately 45 degrees. Chin or forehead down. Soft elbows.

2. Raise arms by squeezing the shoulder blades together. Raise to horizontal, maintain "piper cub" configuration, not "Delta wing". Lower arms slowly and repeat.

2 Sets of 12-15 repetitions.
Beginning weights: 2-5 lbs.

Avoid Pain!

SINGLE ARM ROW

This exercise targets the scapular retractors and part of the latissimus dorsi. This is a very powerful motion for the body, and you may start with 10 to 20 pounds.

Place one knee and shin on the bench. The foot on the floor should be 12 to 18 inches from the bench. Bend forward and support your upper body weight on your arm. Your outside arm should hang straight down. Your support arm, trunk, thigh, and bench should form a rectangle. To maintain good position of the head and neck, look at the bench and not ahead.

With a weight in your outside hand, begin by raising your elbow towards the ceiling. Your arm should remain close to your side, and your forearm should remain vertical throughout the motion. Let your arm slowly return downward, and let the weight pull your shoulder blade down without rotating the trunk. Now repeat the elbow raise. You should feel the work along the lower portion of your shoulder blade. If you are having difficulty isolating the appropriate muscles, begin the elbow raise by moving the elbow towards your hip as you raise it upward. Try not to overuse the biceps. Keeping the forearm vertical will help. Letting your arm rub the side of your body will help reduce the tendency to use the pectoral muscle.

SINGLE ARM ROW

Target: Back

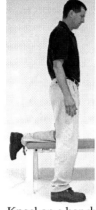

1. Kneel on a bench.

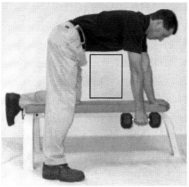

2. Bend forward and support upper body so that a rectangle is formed. Look at the bench. Pick up the weight.

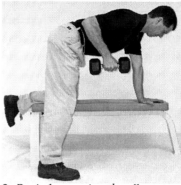

3. Begin by moving the elbow towards the hip,

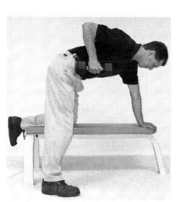

4. then towards the ceiling.

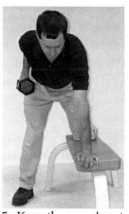

5. Keep the arm close to your side.

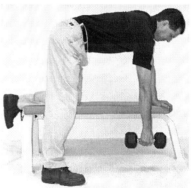

6. Lower the weight towards the floor-- let it stretch the shoulder downward, but don't rotate the trunk. Repeat.

Beginning weight 10-20 lbs.
2 sets of 12-15 repetitions per side.

Avoid Pain!

FRONTAL PULL-DOWN

Pull-down exercises target the latissimus dorsi muscles. This exercise requires a cable machine. Frontal pull-downs are strongly encouraged. Pull-downs behind the head are strongly discouraged because you are not able to keep the ears aligned with the shoulders. Generally start with 20 to 30 pounds of weight.

Begin positioning for the exercise by grabbing the bar with the hands one to two times your shoulder width apart. You may need to experiment to find the best and most comfortable grip width.

Sit down, pulling the bar with you. Lean back from the hips to approximately a 60-degree angle from the bench. Find neutral spine and pelvis by moving back and forth from 12 to 6 o'clock and finding the midpoint between the movements. Align the ears over the shoulders.

Pull the bar down to lightly touch the top of the chest. The cable should be within one inch of your chin. You can imagine your arms sliding down a roof, pulling the bar and cable downward. The work should be felt between the shoulder blades and down to the lower back. Let the bar pull your arms back up to stretch the shoulders, but do not lose the positioning of the trunk. Repeat the pull-down for 12 to 15 repetitions. A version of this exercise can be done with a latex band (p. 107).

FRONTAL PULL-DOWN

Target: Back

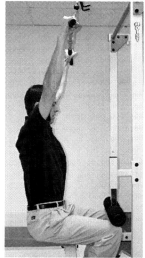

1. Grab bar so that hands are slightly wider than shoulder width, then sit.

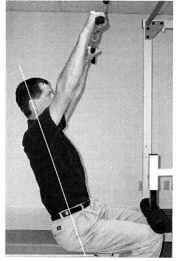

2. Lean the trunk back to 60 degree angle. Neutralize spine and align ears with shoulders.

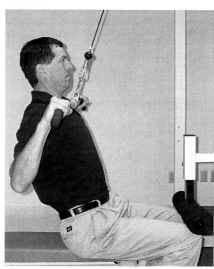

3. Pull the bar downward to the breast bone, just under the chin.

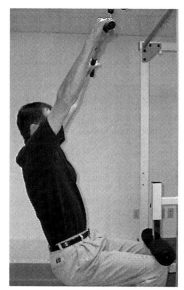

4. Slowly let the bar return up and allow the shoulders to stretch without losing trunk position; repeat pull-down.

Beginning weight 20-30 lbs.
2 sets of 12-15 repetitions.

Avoid Pain!

SEATED ROW

This exercise targets the scapular retractors including the rhomboids, lower and middle trapezius, and possibly some latissimus dorsi. The back extensors are also heavily recruited. Start with 15 to 20 pounds of resistance.

The exercise is generally done sitting flat on the floor, but if correct positioning of the spine cannot be realized because of tight hamstrings, sitting on a short stool or block may help. A cable machine with a low pull is required, although the exercise can be done with a latex band and some imagination.

Sit in front of the machine with your legs straight and your feet braced against the machine. Grab the vertical bars and lean back to approximately a 30-degree angle from the vertical. Find neutral pelvis by moving between 6 o'clock (anterior tilt) and 12 o'clock (posterior tilt). Look straight ahead. Vertical handles or a rope that allows the hands to be vertical seems to work best. The start position is with the elbows straight. Draw the handles back toward the center of your abdomen. Your elbows should move straight back so that your arms stay close to your body. Squeeze the shoulder blades together at the end of the pull.

The work should be felt through the upper back. Slowly release to the start position with the elbows straight and the elbows protracted. Do not let your trunk slump forward. Retract and pull again.

SEATED ROW

Target: Back

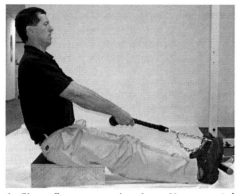 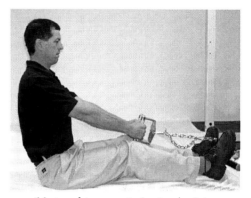

1. Sit on floor or very low box. Knees straight as possible to achieve neutral spine/pelvis.

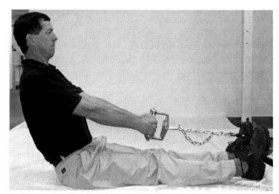 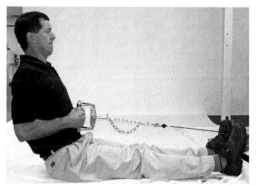

2. Lean back 30 degrees.

3. Pull bar to center of upper abdomen by pulling elbows straight back. Work is felt between shoulder blades.

2 sets of 12-15 repetitions.
Beginning weight of 15-20 lbs.

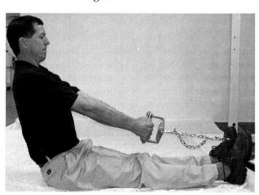

4. Let the weight pull the arms back out to feel some stretch in the shoulders; repeat the exercise.

Avoid Pain!

BENT-OVER ROW

This exercise requires being able to perform a reasonably good wall or Olympic style squat (pp. 48, 44). The target area includes the scapular retractors and all of the spinal extensor muscles of the thoracic and lumbar spine. It may not be a good choice if you have low back problems. Start with 20 to 25 pounds of weight.

The bent-over row can be done with dumbbells, but is probably best done with a bar. Begin with a grip that is one and a half to two times your shoulder width. Move into a good squat position so that your thighs are 30 to 45 degrees from horizontal. Keep your shins vertical and your chest up. Look straight ahead. Now raise the bar towards your upper chest. Your elbows will move towards the ceiling, and your forearms will be as vertical as possible. Your shoulder blades will squeeze together, and the bar should lightly touch your chest. Lower the bar slowly, letting the shoulder blades drop, but do not lose the squat positioning. Repeat the lift.

BENT-OVER ROW
Target: Back

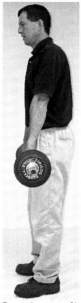

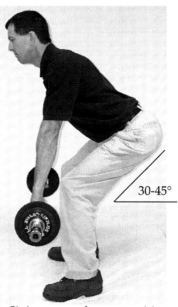

30-45°

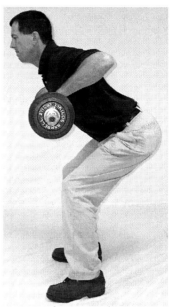

1. Start in standing position holding a bar or dumbbells with wide grip.

2. Sit into a good squat position with thighs 30-45° from horizontal. Shins vertical and chest up.

3a. Pull the bar to the upper chest.

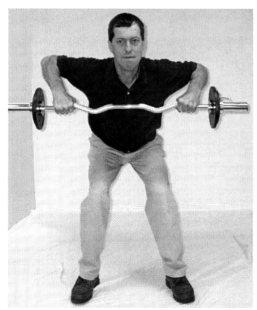

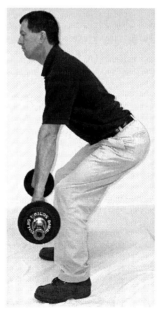

3b. Bar pulled to upper chest.

4. Slowly relax the arms and repeat lifts.

2 sets of 12-15 repetitions.
Begin with 20-25 lbs.

Avoid Pain!

Upper Body Exercises
For The Chest

BENCH FLY

The bench fly is a fairly easy exercise that targets the pectoral or chest muscles. When done correctly, it also provides a stretching component as well. Begin with 3 to 5 pounds of weight in each hand.

Lie on a bench so that your feet are also supported. If the bench is very short, a chair or stool can be used as a foot prop. This exercise can be done on the floor using pillows to elevate the upper body.

Find neutral pelvis by moving back and forth between 6 and 12 o'clock and finding the middle position. The chin is slightly tucked. The arms are now brought up over the chest. Introduce a slight to moderate bend to the elbows to form a "hug a tree" position. Maintain this constant elbow angle throughout repetitions of the exercise.

Let the arms fall straight apart. Avoid any rotation of the shoulders. The arms should remain in an imaginary corridor that would form a straight line through the shoulders and chest. As the arms come to the bottom of the motion, squeeze the shoulder blades together under you. A slight stretch should be felt in the chest muscles. Return to the start position and repeat.

BENCH FLY

Target: Chest

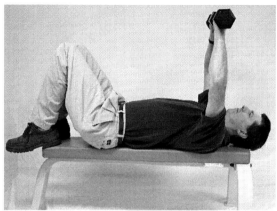

1. Lies with feet on bench. Find neutral pelvis. Hands aligned over chest, chin is slightly tucked.

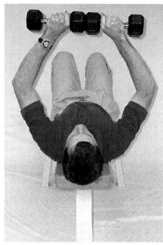

2. Arms in "Hug a Tree" position. Maintain a constant elbow angle.

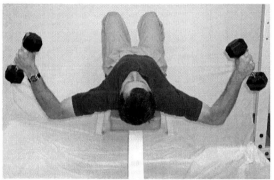

3. Let the arms fall apart. Arms, elbows, and hands move as solid units.

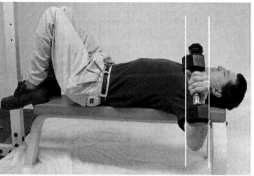

4. Maintain a straight line through hands, elbows, and shoulders. Stay in corridor.

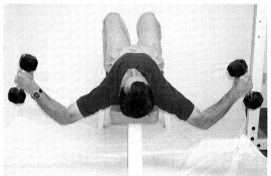

5. Squeeze shoulder blades together at bottom of movement.

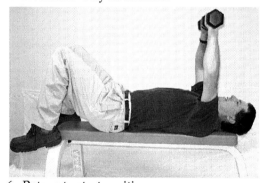

6. Return to start position.

Beginning weight of 3-5 lbs.
2 sets of 12-15 repetitions

Avoid Pain!

INCLINE DUMBBELL PRESS

A dumbbell press has elements in common with both a bench press and a bench fly (pp. 138, 142). You will use slightly more weight than with the fly, but substantially less weight than with the bench press. You will need a 45-degree incline bench. Up to a 60-degree incline will work. Begin with 5 to 8 pounds of weight in each hand.

Lie on the bench with the pelvis in neutral. The elbows will be straight with the weights over your head. To bring the weights down, let your elbows move straight towards the floor, keeping forearms vertical. The end of the weights should rest in the crease where the shoulder and chest muscles meet. Now push the weights back up to the starting position to repeat the exercise.

INCLINE DUMBBELL PRESS

Target: Chest

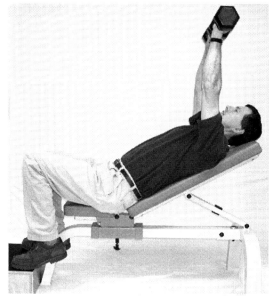

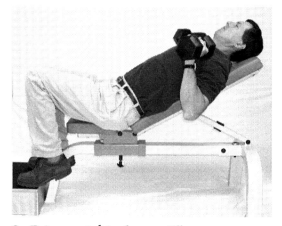

2. Bring weights down. Elbows move straight to floor.

1. Lie on incline bench, arms straight with weight over eyes.

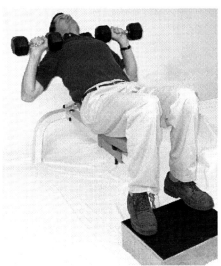

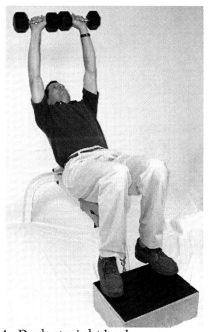

3. Weights will rest in crease between shoulder and chest muscles.

4. Push straight back up over eyes.

2 sets of 12-15 repetitions
Begin with 5-8 lbs.

Avoid Pain!

BENCH PRESS

The bench press allows for much heavier weights to be used than either the bench fly or the dumbbell press (pp. 138, 140). In addition to providing more resistance to strengthen the chest muscles, the extra weight helps to restore backward bend movement to the upper back by flattening it against the bench. A flexed thoracic spine is generally one of the first areas of postural breakdown.

A bench press is best done on a weight bench with a rack system. If you have no experience with this kind of exercise, a knowledgeable helper, called a "spotter," will be necessary. Lie with your feet on the bench and your pelvis in neutral with the chin slightly tucked. Olympic bars, by themselves, weigh 45 pounds. A solid, small diameter bar will weight 20 to 25 pounds, and EZ curl bars will weight anywhere from 15 to 25 pounds. Begin with a total weight of 10 to 20 pounds. Grab the bar so that your hands are 1.5 to 2 times the width of your shoulders.

Unrack the bar and bring it over your upper chest. Keep your wrists in neutral and the bar over your chest throughout the movement. Bring the bar down to your chest, letting the elbows move straight towards the floor. Lightly touch the bar to the breastbone before returning the bar to the start position. Check that the wrists remain in a straight or neutral position. Repeat the bench press.

BENCH PRESS
Target: Chest

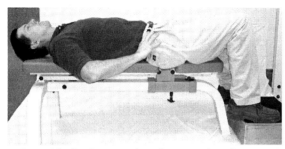

1. Lie with the feet on a bench or stool with neutral pelvis and chin slightly tucked.

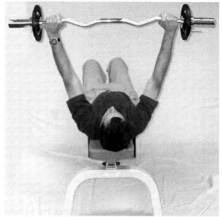

2. Grab the bar 1.5 to 2 x shoulder width.

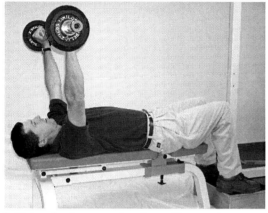

3. Bring the bar over the chest. Keep wrists neutral.

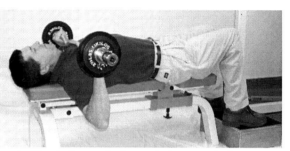

4. Slowly lower the bar to lightly touch the upper chest. Elbows move straight towards the floor.

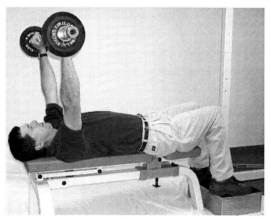

5. Return to the start position.

Beginning weight 10-20 lbs.
2 sets of 12-15 repetitions.

Avoid Pain!

Upper Body Exercises
For The Lateral Shoulders

DOOR FRAME LATERAL RAISE

This exercise targets the deltoid and rotator cuff muscles. The scapular stabilizers and postural muscles will be automatically engaged as soon as you grab the weights. You must therefore try to use optimal positioning with this and any other exercise, especially one that is performed standing, to reinforce good posture.

Begin with your back against a post or door frame. Position the back of your head against the door frame so you're looking straight ahead. Your feet should be 4 to 8 inches from the bottom of the door frame. Find neutral spine and pelvis by moving from a 12 o'clock to 6 o'clock tilt. Do this 3 to 4 times, and then stop with the spine and pelvis at approximately the midpoint of these movements. This should position you fairly close to ideal posture. It will also prevent momentum or alteration of form that would degrade the exercise.

Generally start with 3 to 5 pounds of weight in each hand. Begin the lateral raise portion of the exercise with the arms at your sides with the palms facing in and the thumb side of the hand aiming forward. Raise the arms straight out from your sides. The arms will rotate so that when horizontal, the palms will face forward and the thumb side of the hands will aim toward the ceiling. Keep the elbows soft, not locked. Do not allow them to bend to a significant degree. Slowly lower the arms, rotating them back to their starting point. Repeat the lateral raise. Raise only to horizontal with each arm. Remember to maintain the postural alignment throughout your 12 to 15 repetitions.

DOOR FRAME LATERAL RAISE

Target: Lateral Shoulders

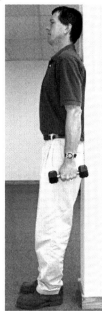

1. Stand with feet 4-8" from a doorframe. Look straight ahead with back of head against the doorframe. Start with neutral pelvis.

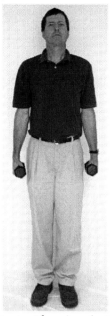

2. Start with palms facing inward.

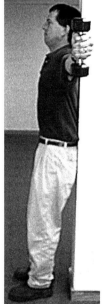

3. Raise arms straight out from sides. Rotate palms forward as the arms come to horizontal.

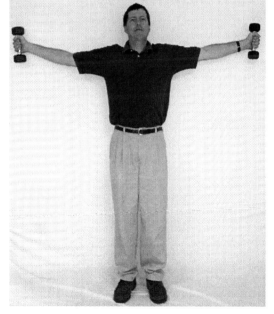

4. Keep elbows soft. Slowly lower to sides and derotate to starting position and repeat.

Beginning weights 3-5 lbs.
2 sets of 12-15 repetitions

Avoid Pain!

147

UPRIGHT ROW

This exercise targets the lateral deltoid, rotator cuff, and the upper trapezius region. The biceps may be recruited to some degree. The motion used with this exercise is similar to the proper way to lift a suitcase or groceries out of the trunk of an automobile. Begin with 15 to 20 pounds of weight.

Like the lateral raise, this exercise is done with your back up to a door frame or post. Hold your spine and pelvis in a neutral position. Your feet should be 4 to 8 inches from the bottom of the door frame, with the back of your head touching the door frame. Your head should be level so you're looking straight forward. Hold a dumbbell weight or bar by its center in front of you with the elbows straight.

Do the "row" by raising the weight straight up. Begin by moving the elbows upward. Keep the weight as close to the body as possible, and raise the bar or weight to collarbone height. Lower the weight slowly, and repeat the lift.

UPRIGHT ROW

Target: Lateral Shoulders

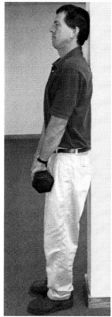

1. Stand with feet 4-8" from a doorframe. Look straight ahead with back of head against the doorframe. Establish neutral pelvis.

2. Grab the weight or bar in the center.

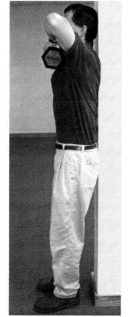

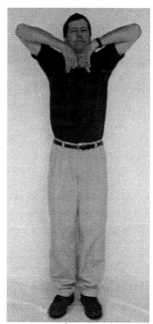

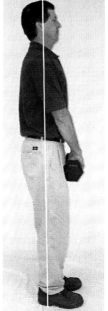

3a. Lift by moving the elbows up.

3b. Pull the weight to collar bone height.

4. Lower slowly and repeat.

Beginning weights 15-20 lbs.
2 sets of 12 to 15 repetitions.

Avoid Pain!

INCLINE LATERAL RAISE

The alternative lateral shoulder exercise is done in an inclined side-lying position.

Start with 3 to 5 pounds. Use an incline bench set at a 30 to 45 degree angle. Position yourself on the incline bench in a side-lying position. Support your head on the downside arm. The other arm holds a weight palm down on the top hipbone. The pelvis is generally in neutral.

Raise the arm as a unit, keeping the palm facing downward and elbow soft. Maximum motion is 90 to 100 degrees from the side of the body. Try to avoid any rotation in the shoulder. Slowly lower the weight to lightly touch the hipbone, and repeat the lift.

This exercise can be done without a bench by leaning over the arm of an overstuffed chair or sitting sideways in a recliner.

INCLINE LATERAL RAISE
Target: Lateral Shoulders

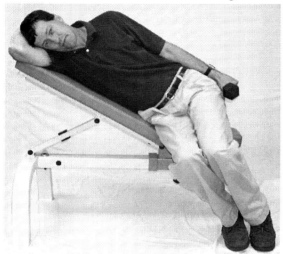

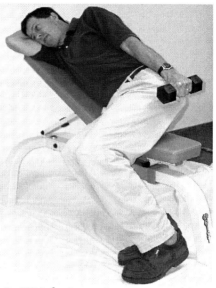

1. Lie on your side on 45° incline bench. Head is supported on the inside arm.

2. Weight is resting on your hip with palm facing downward.

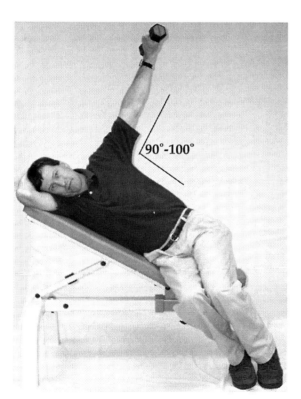

90°-100°

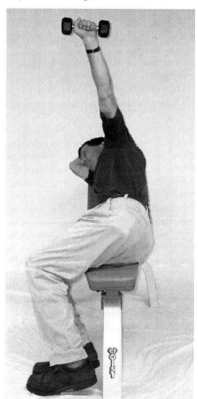

3. Raise the weight to 90° to 100° from the body. Keep the palm facing downward and elbow soft.

4. Keep the arm aligned with the hip. Lower slowly and repeat.

Beginning weight 3-5 lbs.
2 sets of 12-15 repetitions per side

Avoid Pain!

FRONTAL RAISES/BICEP CURLS

A variation on the doorframe exercise will strengthen the muscles in the front of the shoulder.

Start with 3 to 5 pounds of weight in each hand. Position yourself in a door frame or with your back against the upright of an exercise machine, just as for the upright row and lateral raises. Standing biceps curls may also be done with door frame support.

With your pelvis and spine in neutral and your head against the door frame, alternately raise one arm at a time to a 90-degree position. Keep the palms facing downward and the elbows not locked. Allow one arm to finish movement before the other is started.

Bicep curls are executed by bending at the elbow only. Start with 5 to 8 pounds of weight in each hand. Keep your upper arm at your side and bend one elbow only. Rotate your forearm so that the palm faces the shoulder when the elbow is fully bent. Straighten the elbow slowly, and repeat the exercise with the other arm.

FRONTAL RAISES/BICEP CURLS

Target: Front Shoulder Muscles

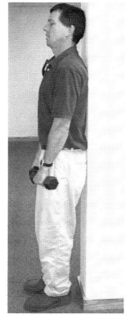 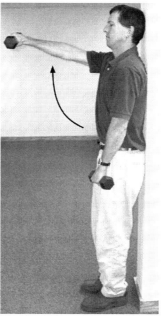

1. Neutral pelvis. Raise one arm at a time to 90°.

2. Keep elbows soft and palms down.

Bicep Curls

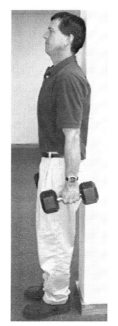 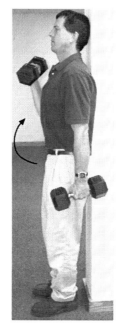

Bend elbows one at a time.

Bend elbows one at a time.
Keep the upper arm stationary.
2 sets of 12–15 repetitions per arm.
Start with 3–5 lbs. for frontal raises and 5–8 lbs. for bicep curls.

Avoid Pain!

Exercises for the Serratus Anterior, Triceps, and Biceps

SUPINE ELBOW EXTENSION

The serratus anterior is a large flat muscle that attaches along the side of the rib cage below the arm pit and runs around the back of the rib cage, under the shoulder blade, to attach along the front inside edge of the shoulder blade. This muscle pulls the shoulder blade forward and tilts it upward to place the ball and socket with its attending rotator cuff muscles in an optimal position to work. Poor functioning of the serratus anterior means that the rotator cuff has to work a little harder every time you move your arm. Inhibition of the serratus anterior is generally the result of poor posture and all its encompassing problems.

The serratus anterior muscle is one of the most neglected muscles in the upper body. Insufficient functioning of this muscle is probably responsible for a great many rotator cuff tears and inflammation of the tendons (tendonitis) and bursa (bursitis) of the shoulder.

The supine elbow extension exercise may help retrain a poorly operating serratus anterior.

Start with 2 to 3 pounds of weight. Lie on a bench with your feet supported. If you are doing this exercise at home, position yourself across the bed or on a couch so that your arm will hang over the edge.

Bring one upper arm to a position beside your head and even with your eye. Bend the elbow in a loose position, letting it hang straight down over the edge of the bench or bed. Stabilize the upper arm in this position by monitoring and/or holding it with the opposite hand. Slowly extend the elbow to a gently locked position, and then slowly let it bend to return to its start position. Work is generally felt along the triceps into the outside edge of the shoulder blade below the armpit.

If pain or a pinching sensation occurs in the top of the shoulder, move the upper arm to a position even with your chin and repeat the exercise. Keep the upper arm absolutely stationary while the forearm is moving. The arm should also be vertical if viewed from the top. If not vertical, the weight tends to end up behind the head in the start position. Generally keep the elbow pointed straight towards the ceiling.

As the exercise gets easier, the upper arm will be positioned closer to horizontal to provide more activation of the serratus anterior.

SUPINE ELBOW EXTENSION

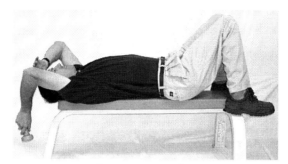

1. Lie on a bench, bed, or couch so your arm can hang over your head.

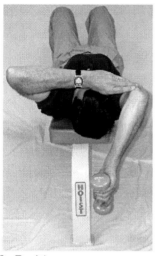

2. Position your upper arm beside your head as close to horizontal as is comfortable. Start even with your eye.

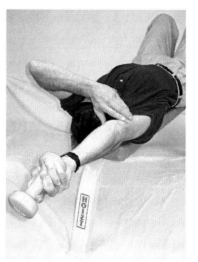

3. Straighten your elbow while keeping your upper arm stationary. Use your opposite hand to stabilize the upper arm.

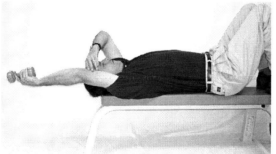

4. Adjust your arm position to relieve pain in the tip of the shoulder or to optimize work in the triceps and shoulder blade areas.

Do 2-3 sets of 10 repetitions.
Start with 2-3 lbs.

Avoid Pain!

INCLINE BICEP CURL

Incline biceps curls work to strengthen the biceps as well as provide a stretch for the chest and shoulders. Generally start with 5 to 8 pounds.

Lie on a 45-degree incline bench with the pelvis in neutral and the chin slightly tucked. Your arms will hang straight down beside the bench with elbows straight. Alternately bend the elbows, keeping the upper arm stationary, raising the weight to your chest. Move only one arm at a time.

INCLINE BICEP CURL

Target: Biceps

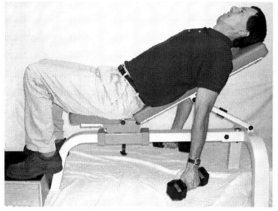

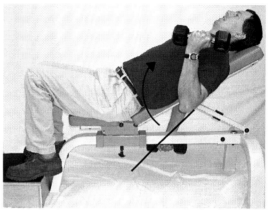

1. Lie on a 45° incline bench with pelvis neutral, chin slightly tucked, and arms hanging down.

2. Alternately bend at the elbows. Keep the upper arm stationary.

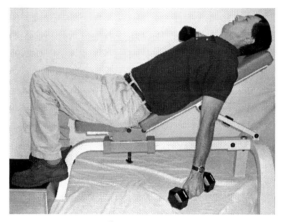

3. Repeat on other side.

Beginning weight of 5 to 8 lbs.
2 sets of 12-15 repetitions.

Avoid Pain!

VII
Foam Roller Exercises

FOAM ROLLER STRETCH
LENGTHWISE VERSION

A 36" x 6" foam roller is a wonderful tool for loosening the spine and for providing a massage to the back muscles. There are two basic techniques that, once mastered, can be modified to suit individual needs.

The lengthwise version is started by lying on a foam roller so you are supported from your tailbone to your head. Bend your knees so your feet are flat and 12 to 18 inches apart. Relax for a few seconds in this position with your arms resting on the floor at your sides.

Now perform a moderate 12 o'clock tilt, slightly tuck your chin, and raise your arms over your head, keeping your elbows almost straight. You should feel a comfortable stretch through the arms and sides of the rib cage. Limit your motion if pain occurs in the top of the shoulders. Moving the arms farther apart may also alleviate discomfort. Hold the stretch for 15 to 20 seconds.

To position for the diagonal stretch, first stabilize your trunk on the roller by resting your arms on the floor at your sides. Shift your hips to one side of the roller so that one side of your pelvis is on the roller and the other side is off the roller. Straighten the knee of the off leg. Move your shoulders so they are shifted slightly to the other side. Rest your head against the side of the roller. Raise your arms over your head. Adjust your right, left, and diagonal positioning so that you are perfectly balanced and draped across the roller. Hold this position for 15 to 20 seconds. Bring your arms back, move to the center position, and repeat the stretch on the opposite diagonal. If these stretches feel good, they can be repeated several times per session and several times per day.

FOAM ROLLER STRETCH
LENGTHWISE VERSION

For Straight Position

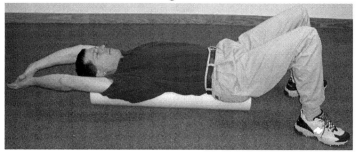

Chin tucked and tummy tight.

For Diagonal Position

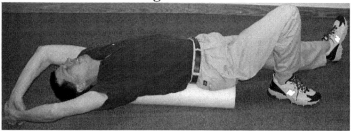

Drape body over roller.
Find relaxed position

Head beside roller

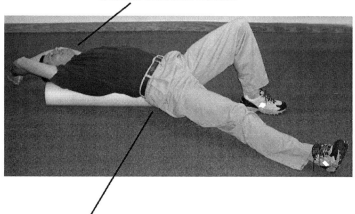

Opposite hip off with knee straight.

15-20 seconds per position
Repeat 1-3 times each side

Avoid Pain!

FOAM ROLLER
CROSSWISE VERSION

This version of the foam roller exercise is generally good for improving backward bending mobility of the thoracic spine.

Start by sitting on the floor and leaning back over a 36" by 6" foam roller so that it's positioned across the lower part of your shoulder blades. Lace your fingers behind your head and point your elbows toward the ceiling so your forearms are touching the sides of your head. Bend your knees and position your feet flat on the floor so they are 12 to 18 inches apart.

Lift your bottom off the floor into a bridge position. Let your head down so you are looking straight at the ceiling. Now pull with your legs to move the roller slowly to the top of your shoulder blades. You may need to lift your bottom up a little higher if you feel the roller sliding out from under you. Now slowly push with your legs to move the roller down to the bottom of your rib cage. You may need to lower your bottom to keep your trunk parallel to the floor. If you get the roller too low on your back, the pressure may be uncomfortable. Generally do not go below rib cage level. Repeat the rolling motion and return the roller to the top of your shoulders. This can be done 8 to 10 times.

Then do the rolling technique at slight angles. Move your feet 2 steps to the right. Repeat the rolling motion described above 8 to 10 times. Now move your feet 2 steps to the left of center and repeat the movement.

If you find that the roller is too uncomfortable or too hard, place a folded towel or long flat pillow between you and the roller. You can also roll yourself up and down on the roller by sliding your bottom along the floor. This will reduce the pressure applied to the back and make the exercise more comfortable. See the next exercise.

FOAM ROLLER
CROSSWISE VERSION

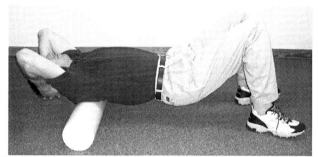
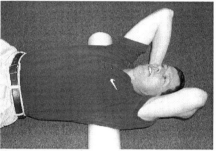

Look at ceiling and support your head. Body parallel to floor.

Do not go above top or below bottom of your rib cage.

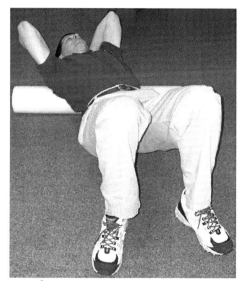
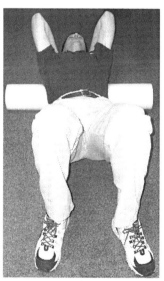

Slight angle of body.

Body straight on roller.

8-10 rolls with body straight.
8-10 rolls with slight angle of your body.
8-10 rolls at other angle.

Avoid Pain!

FOAM ROLLER
BOTTOM DOWN AND PILLOW VARIATION

If your spine seems too tender to tolerate the pressure of the foam roller, these two techniques may help.

The first is keeping your bottom in contact with the floor as you roll from shoulder to lower thoracic spine. Another technique would be to place a folded towel or long flat pillow between your back and the roller. If needed, these two techniques can be combined.

In both techniques, you still use your arms to support your head. Look towards the ceiling to maintain good head and neck alignment. Roll back and forth 6 to 8 times, both straight and at slight angles.

FOAM ROLLER
BOTTOM DOWN AND PILLOW VARIATION

Bottom Down

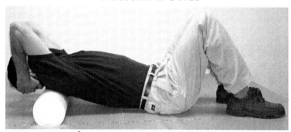

1. Support head and lean back to contact roller.

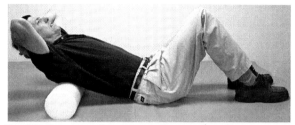

2. Slide your bottom along the floor to move the roller to the top of the shoulders.

Pillow

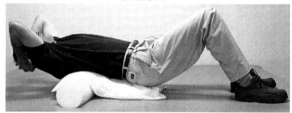

1. Place a folded towel or long flat pillow between you and the roller.

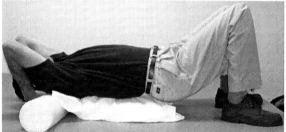

2. Use the same rolling technique as described above.

Look at the ceiling. Feel forearms close to head to keep shoulder blades protracted. 6-8 rolls straight and on each diagonal.

Avoid Pain!

FOAM ROLLER
HEAD OFF END TECHNIQUE

This technique is helpful if the very top of the thoracic spine is restricted in backward bending movement. A "hump" can develop at the base of the neck. Care must be taken with this exercise so as not to over-extend the neck.

Lie on the foam roller lengthwise. Identify the spinous processes of the 7th cervical and 1st thoracic vertebrae with your fingertips. These are the first big bony bumps at the center of the base of your neck. Move yourself on the foam roller until the edge of the roller is 1/2 to 3/4 of an inch below the 1st thoracic vertebra. Lace your fingers together and hold your head. Move the pelvis and lumbar spine into a 12 o'clock or posterior tilt. Tuck the chin slightly and let your head and neck move towards the floor. Keep the head in a retracted position and level. This should provide a feeling of pressure or stretch in the spine near the edge of the roller. Try slightly rotating the head to one side or the other to find the most restricted spot. Work 15 to 20 seconds at this level. It may be helpful to pull the head away from the shoulders to provide a traction force through the neck. The traction may enhance the movement in the tight areas.

Move your body up the roller by 1/2 to 3/4 of an inch. The roller should now be 1/2 to 3/4 of an inch lower on your spine. Retighten the 12 o'clock tilt, retuck the chin, and let the head retract again. Play with positioning from one side to the other. You can repeat this technique through the top 4 to 5 inches of the thoracic spine.

FOAM ROLLER
HEAD OFF END TECHNIQUE

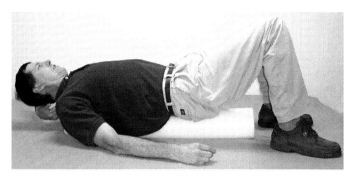

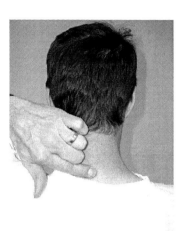

1. Lie on roller. Find largest bumps at base of neck, the spinous processes of C7 and T1. Slide up the roller so that the edge of the roller is 1/2"-3/4 " below the bumps. Support the head.

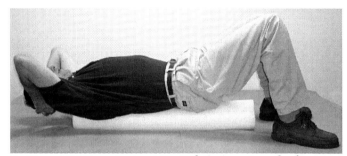

2. Do a 12:00 posterior tilt. While keeping the head level, let it sink toward the floor.

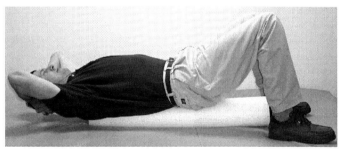

3. Hold the position for 15-20 seconds. Stretch should be felt in the space at the edge of the roller. Move slightly to the right or left and hold again. Move 1/2"-3/4" up the roller and repeat. Only work within 4-5" below the C7/T1 bumps.

Avoid Pain!

FOAM ROLLER
LUMBAR SPINE TECHNIQUE

This technique may be good for you if there are extension restrictions in the lowest part of the lumbar spine, or if you tend to have a very flat spine.

Sit on the floor. Pull the roller up to the base of your spine. Hold the roller as you lean back over it. Resting the forearms on the roller may be more comfortable. Gently roll back and forth over the roller to nudge the spine into more backward bending. Repeat 8 to 10 rolls, or bend backward over a tight spot and hold the position for 15 to 20 seconds.

FOAM ROLLER
LUMBAR SPINE TECHNIQUE

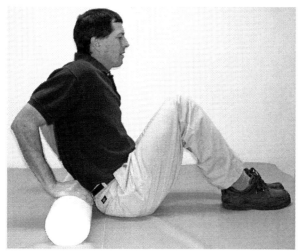

1. Pull the roller tight against the pelvis.

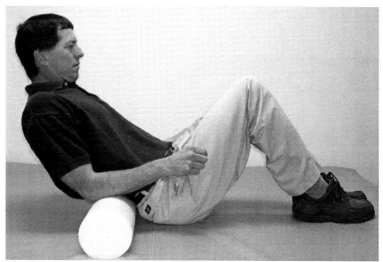

2. Rest forearms on the roller . Move up and down the roller with small movement on the lumbar spine.

Repeat 8-10 repetitions or hold 15-20 seconds.

Avoid Pain!

FOAM ROLLER
MID-THORACIC SPINE TECHNIQUE

Persistent extension restrictions in the mid- and upper-thoracic spine can be addressed with this technique.

Lie on the roller at a large enough angle so the shoulder blades straddle the roller. Lace your fingers to support the head. Point your elbows toward the ceiling so your forearms hug the side of your head.

Roll across the roller from one shoulder blade to the other. Try to let your spine drape over the roller as you move. Move slowly across the roller for 8 to 10 repetitions on each angle.

FOAM ROLLER
MID-THORACIC SPINE TECHNIQUE

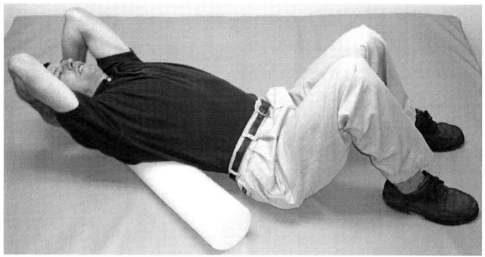

1. Adjust to a large angle with the roller in the center of the thoracic spine.

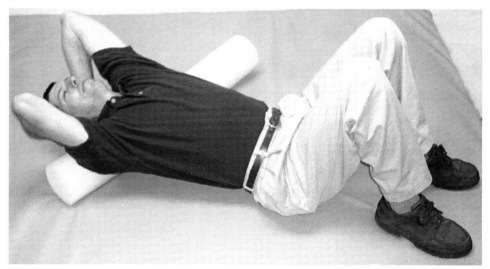

2. Work on the other side. Roller is straddled by shoulder blades.

Look at the ceiling. Keep forearms close to
head to keep shoulder blades protracted.
8-10 rolls on each diagonal.

Avoid Pain!

9
Case Studies

The patients depicted in these summaries represent people who had problems associated with breakdown of the musculoskeletal system. Manual therapy and other pain relievers (*i.e.* ultrasound, hot and cold packs, and electrical stimulation) were used with most of the patients. All of the patients were instructed to avoid pain with all of their activities, including their exercises.

PATIENT NO. 1: NECK AND SHOULDER PAIN

A 65-year-old man described a two- to three-month history of neck and shoulder pain. The problems had not resolved with rest and medication. He said that pain was now starting in the upper arm.

He had extremely poor posture. He had a bent and rigid upper back that placed his head in a very protracted position in front of his shoulders. He could not lie flat on a firm treatment table and have his head touch the table. The muscles in the front of his chest were extremely tight, restricting overall shoulder motion. Motion of the head and neck was limited and painful in almost all directions. Mechanical dysfunction was found and treated in the thoracic spine and rib cage. The patient began a home exercise program.

Because of the severity of the patient's postural problems, the exercises were modified for comfort and effectiveness. The play dead and supine attention exercises were done with his head on a folded bath towel. The towel was thick enough to allow his head to stay level when he was lying flat on his back. The towel roll exercise was started with a single towel placed under the center of the spine and enough support under the head to allow the head to stay level. The upper arm would only flex to 135 degrees (180 degrees is considered optimal). The wall angel was done sitting and without the arm component. The patient could not move his head within two inches of the wall. The patient was also given the arm stretch to improve mobility across the chest musculature.

On subsequent visits, manual therapy techniques were used with good success. But their benefit would have been extremely limited if the patient did not continue his home exercises.

No changes were made with the home program on the second visit. By the third visit, we were able to reduce the thickness of the towels under the head with the attention, play dead, and towel roll exercises. A significant reduction in pain was noted.

The fifth and final visit was three weeks after the patient's initial session. Even though his posture was not perfect, military, ramrod straight, it was much better than what we started with. The patient could lie flat on his back comfortably without any support under his head. He could raise his arms to approximately 160 degrees when doing the towel roll stretch. He was doing this exercise with two towels placed under the center of his back. He could do the wall angel standing (with knees bent) with the head on the wall and the arms raised to 140 degrees.

The patient was discharged with the recommendation that he continue with his exercises on a daily basis.

PATIENT NO. 2: NECK AND ARM PAIN

A 55-year-old University professor described a one-year history of neck, right shoulder, and arm pain. The arm pain would radiate down to the elbow.

She had extremely poor posture with the mid and upper portion of the thoracic spine being very flexed, causing fairly severe protraction of the head and neck or forward head posture. The low back was fairly flat. A moderate amount of mechanical dysfunction was found in the thoracic spine and rib cage. Mild problems were found in the neck. Movement of the head and neck caused mild pain in the neck. There was radiation of pain down the right arm with right rotation and/or side bending. There was essentially no motion of the upper back with movement of the head and neck, indicating a "kink" in the system.

There was very poor strength and recruitment in the postural muscles throughout the neck and upper back. The muscles that control the shoulder blade were very weak. She had substantial difficulty isolating the pelvic clock muscles in both the six and twelve o'clock directions.

The patient began a home exercise program. The play dead was begun with the patient flat (no towel under the shoulders). She was given the supine attention exercise. Lying on the towel roll felt good, but the patient could only use a single towel. She could flex the shoulders to only 140 degrees (180 degrees is considered optimal). The thumbs were pointed down to the floor to alleviate shoulder discomfort with this exercise. The wall angel was done sitting with the arms raised 45 degrees above the horizontal.

Five days later, the patient noted substantial improvement. Her home exercise program was reviewed and upgraded to include using a folded bath towel under her shoulders with the play dead exercise. She could also add another towel with the towel roll exercise.

A week later, the patient reported continued improvements. She was instructed in the basic techniques for using a foam roller. The wall angel was upgraded to the standing version. The other exercises were still challenging, and we left them as they were.

The patient's next visit was three weeks after her initial session. She noted discomfort only after walking her dog (who pulled on the leash) and working out on the same day. That session included an overview of upper body exercises. We included the supine elbow extension exercise to specifically target the serratus anterior. Good activation of the muscle was noted with the upper arm positioned at a 135-degree angle. Impingement in the shoulders would occur with increased flexion. The foam roller exercise was modified to add a flat pillow over the foam roller because of tenderness in the spine.

The following week, the patient was doing extremely well. We made minor corrections to her upper body exercises and added reverse and side step lunges. She also learned supine heel touch downs for abdominal strengthening. All of the areas were recruited well, but fatigued very rapidly.

The patient's final visit was five weeks after her initial session. She reported complete resolution of her original pain. She had occasional upper back and shoulder fatigue with sustained kitchen activities. A review of her exercises showed good technique. We added a narrow-based wall squat to further improve the mobility in her spine. The patient was discharged after this visit.

PATIENT NO. 3: LOW BACK PAIN

A 49-year-old woman described a 12-month history of worsening back pain. At the time of the evaluation, she rated her pain as severe. The pain was generally localized to the left lower back area. Bending or prolonged standing activities would worsen her problems. She would be uncomfortable after lying in bed for more than six hours. She was very uncomfortable when first getting out of bed in the morning.

Her posture was not too bad, with only mild protraction of the head and neck over a mildly increased forward bend in the upper back. Major mechanical dysfunction was found and treated in the pelvic region. Her hip abductors and extensors were extremely weak and very poorly recruited. The 12 o'clock portion of the pelvic clock was very weak and poorly isolated. The piriformis musculature was very tight bilaterally. Overall trunk range of motion was only mildly limited. There was too much movement in the lower lumbar spine with backward bending, indicating poor backward bend movement through the pelvis and upper back.

We began her home program with supine gluteal retraining, clam, pelvic clock, piriformis stretch, and the wall angel. The wall angel was fairly easy, but the other exercises required a great deal of concentration and effort.

One week later, the patient was able to upgrade the home exercise program to include prone gluteal retraining instead of the supine version. We also added the door frame backward bend exercise to help improve motion of the sacrum. The patient was instructed in the basic techniques for the foam roller to help improve backward bend through the thoracic spine.

By the fourth week, the patient had sufficient strength and recruitment in the gluteal musculature that we were able to add the reverse and side step lunges. We deleted the clam and gluteal retraining. The wall squat was also added to further promote active control of extension through the thoracic spine. The patient reported a mild improvement in her back pain.

Good overall progress was being made by the fifth visit. The thoracic spine was somewhat tender after a weekend trip, and she learned how to use a pillow over the foam roller to make the exercise more comfortable.

By the seventh week, the patient reported that she had been pain free for ten days. Her exercises were reviewed and upgraded to include supine heel touch downs for abdominal strengthening.

The patient's final visit came nine weeks after her initial session. She reported only very mild intermittent problems with pain, and these occurred only after strenuous physical activity. With this session, we reviewed her current exercises that included reverse and side step lunges, advanced abdominal exercises, piriformis stretching, and the wall angel. At the patient's request, she was shown a basic upper body exercise program that she could follow at home. She was advised to continue with all of her exercises on a three day per week maintenance schedule.

PATIENT NO. 4: LOW BACK PAIN

A 35-year-old man had been suffering with low back pain for several years. He was usually better in the morning than in the evening. Three to four hours of sitting would give him severe pain. He was beginning to have intermittent leg pain. Yard and housework would trigger severe bouts of back pain that would last for several days. He had been through other conservative treatments including anti-inflammatory medication, muscle relaxants, extension exercises, and even an epidural injection.

His initial assessment revealed fairly poor posture with protraction of the head and shoulders, and was a moderate increase in the thoracic kyphosis. His low back tended to be flat despite his continued good compliance with his extension exercises. Trunk range of motion was fairly good with mild pain elicited at the end ranges of movement. Shallow single leg wall squats were very unsteady, indicating weakness in the hip musculature. Moderate mechanical dysfunction was found in the spine and pelvis. Very poor strength and recruitment were found in the hip abductors and extensors. The left side was worse than the right. He had reasonably good control of the abdominal musculature. Hip mobility was fairly good except for moderately tight piriformis musculature.

During the initial session, the patient was instructed in the pelvic clock, wall angel, prone gluteal retraining, clam exercise, and piriformis stretch. The clock was fairly easy. Some difficulty was found with the clam and gluteal retraining. The wall angel was very difficult. The piriformis stretch felt good.

One week later, substantial improvement was noted by the patient with his second visit. We were able to upgrade his home program to include the supine heel touch down for abdominal strengthening. We attempted the side step lunge for closed chain recruitment of the hip abductors, but he was unable to hit the target. He was able to do a single leg door frame squat with good recruitment of the muscle behind the hip bone (hip abductors). The gluteus maximus was activated well with the reverse step lunge. A narrow-based wall squat was used to promote improved backward bending through the upper lumbar and thoracic spine. Slight abdominal tension relieved discomfort in the low back with this exercise.

The patient's third visit came three weeks after his initial session. He noted mild soreness in the gluteal musculature. We reviewed his exercises, and he demonstrated difficulty with the single leg door frame squat. We tried the ball on the wall exercise, which worked fairly well. Once the hip abductors were found with this exercise, the patient was then able to accurately do the side step lunge. A correction was made to the reverse step lunge that involved stabilizing the lower portion of the stance leg to reduce unnecessary motion. He was instructed in the basic foam roller exercises for improving motion in the thoracic spine.

The patient's final visit was four weeks after his initial session. He was happy to report complete resolution of his back pain. His posture had substantially improved and he demonstrated very good recruitment and strength in the supportive musculature in the trunk and the pelvis. We concluded our session with an overview of upper body exercises and the patient was discharged.

I have spoken with this patient several times in the past year, and he continues to do well. He notes that if he slacks off on his exercises, he experiences some return of his pain. The pain will go away when he resumes his exercises.

PATIENT NO. 5: KNEE PAIN

A 40-year-old woman told of several months of worsening knee pain. Kneeling and descending stairs had become painful. This pain had forced her to curtail her weekly volleyball games. Her medical history included arthroscopic surgery on this knee for torn cartilage five years earlier.

An inspection of the knee revealed very little swelling. Tests for loose or lax ligaments and cartilage tears revealed no problems. Kneecap stability and tracking were good. She had full knee range of motion, and the strength in the quadriceps and hamstrings was very good. Flexibility in the lateral thigh, hamstrings, and quadriceps was reasonably good. Moderate tightness was found in the piriformis musculature. She had moderately poor posture. Strength and isolated recruitment in the hip abductors and extensors were very poor. The abdominal muscles were very poorly controlled and weak. There was a strong tendency to push with the legs when attempting the 12:00 tilt. Shallow single leg squats were very unsteady and mildly painful in the right knee.

A home program began with prone gluteal retraining, clam, pelvic clock, piriformis stretching, and the seated wall angel. The patient was unable to do the standing version of the wall angel. The lie down exercises were to be done twice a day, and the wall angel was to be done five or six times during the day.

Ten days after her initial session, she reported mild improvement in her knee pain. Her exercises were reviewed, and only minor corrections were needed. She was able to graduate to the standing version of the wall angel.

Three weeks after her initial session, the patient noted continued gradual improvement. She noted that the exercises had become fairly easy. She was instructed in the reverse and side step lunges as well as a narrow-based wall squat. She was able to do these well and without knee pain. The clam and prone gluteal retraining were deleted from her program.

Five weeks after her initial session, the patient noted knee pain only if the knee was pushed into hyperextension. The exercises were going extremely well. She was given the supine heel touch down for advanced abdominal strengthening. We looked at the bench fly, seated reverse fly, and door frame lateral raises for upper body exercises.

The patient's final visit came eight weeks after her initial session. She reported almost complete resolution of her knee pain. She was shown bench press, frontal pull down, and incline reverse fly exercises. She was to add weight to the reverse and side step lunges, and continue with all of the exercises on a three-day-per-week basis.

The patient was seen informally three months after her last treatment session, and she reported her knee pain had completely resolved and not returned.

PATIENT NO. 6: PLANTAR FASCIITIS

The plantar fascia is a structure on the bottom of the foot that attaches from the heel bone and fans out to attach to the base of the toes to help maintain the arches in the bottom of the foot. If it becomes overloaded, pain and inflammation can result. This patient had been dealing with worsening plantar fasciitis for several years.

The patient was a 45-year-old female secretary who experienced severe pain in the bottom of both feet, especially first thing in the morning. The pain would improve as she walked about, but would worsen if she stood or walked for more than 20 minutes. Oral medication, splints, taping, and orthotics seemed to provide only marginal benefit.

An evaluation revealed that the plantar surface of the foot was fairly tender. Her posture was not too bad except for a tendency to stand with her body tipped forward so that her body weight shifted to the balls of the feet. Shallow single leg door frame squats were extremely unsteady. The hips were fairly restricted in the piriformis musculature. There was moderate tightness through the front of the thigh including the hip flexors. Internal rotation was very limited in the left hip, but not so much in the right. The supportive musculature in the trunk and the pelvis was very weak and very poorly re-cruited.

The patient's home exercise program consisted of the standard wall angel, postural cueing, pelvic clock, clam, prone gluteal retraining, and the piriformis stretch. Prone gluteal retraining, clam, and pelvic clock were difficult to recruit. The wall angel was done standing, but the arms could only be rotated to 45 degrees upward because of poor abdominal control. She felt very awkward with the postural cueing exercise.

The following week, she reported less morning pain. Minor corrections were made to the exercises. Manual therapy was used to improve mobility in the left hip, and stretching was applied to the piriformis musculature.

Two weeks after her initial session, the patient reported substantial improvement. She was able to stand and walk in the morning without extreme pain. The reverse and side step lunges were added to her home program to replace the clam and gluteal retrain-ing. Rapid fatigue of the musculature was noted in the closed chain mode. The patient was also shown the standing hip flexor stretch.

During the third week after the initial session, the foot pain continued to lessen. Minor corrections were made to the reverse and side step lunges. Deep massage and ultrasound were used over the plantar surfaces of both feet. This significantly reduced the tenderness over the plantar fascia.

The patient's final visit came four weeks after the initial session. She reported mini-mal pain through the morning and drastic improvements in her comfort with walking. Now when standing, most of her weight was carried over the ankles instead of over the balls of the feet. The patient's exercise program was reviewed, and she was discharged.

PATIENT NO. 7: KNEE PAIN

Knee pain is often addressed with strengthening and stretching of the quadriceps and hamstrings. Sometimes the pain will be alleviated. If problems persist when strength and mobility of the hamstrings and quadriceps are optimized, then the problem must lie elsewhere.

A 16-year-old female soccer player described a one-year history of bilateral knee pain. The right side tended to be worse than the left. MRI's and X-ray studies were negative. Previous physical therapy aimed at the quadriceps and hamstrings was ineffective. She rated her knee pain at 8/10 after her soccer games.

Her initial evaluation revealed good strength and mobility in the hamstrings and quadriceps. There was very mild swelling along the joint line of both knees. Tests for loose and lax ligaments and cartilage tears revealed no problem. She had mild postural deficits with some protraction of the head and neck, some increase in the bend in the upper back, and a mild increase in sway to the lower back. The piriformis muscles were moderately tight on both sides. Recruitment and strength were extremely poor throughout the trunk and the pelvis. With instruction in her home exercises, we found that there was almost no isolated recruitment of the gluteus maximus. Retraining began with the supine version of gluteal retraining. Hip abduction was extremely weak and difficult to isolate with the clam exercise. The pelvic clock exercise was started. Six o'clock was fairly easy. The abdominal musculature was extremely difficult to isolate in the twelve o'clock direction. The wall angel was moderately difficult.

On the patient's second visit, very mild improvement was reported with regards to knee pain. The exercise program was reviewed, and the supine gluteal retraining exercise was upgraded to the prone version.

The third visit came two weeks after the patient's initial session. We attempted to upgrade to the closed chain exercises, but found that recruitment was not yet adequate. The patient continued with the clam and prone gluteal retraining. We were able to add the supine heel touch down for abdominal strengthening.

On her fourth visit three weeks after her initial session, she reported continuing lessening of her knee pain. At this time, she was able to recruit the hip abductors with the side step lunge, and the hip extensors with the reverse step lunge. Rapid fatigue was reported once the musculature was isolated. She was to continue with the wall angel, piriformis stretch, and abdominal strengthening.

The patient's final visit came five weeks after her initial session. She had experienced only very mild knee discomfort after playing soccer in a weekend tournament. We reviewed her exercises and made only minor corrections to the reverse step lunge. We added the standing hip flexor stretch because of mild tightness through the front of the thigh musculature. The patient was then discharged from physical therapy.

The patient's mother stopped by our office three weeks after the patient's last session. She reported that the knee pain had not reoccurred and that the patient was able to play soccer without problems.